7-minute Chair Yoga for Fibromyalgia

Lose weight, relief pain and feel better

First Edition

Table of Content

Introduction

Allow me to draw you into the profound "Mindful Movement" world through a captivating narrative—a testament to the transformative power of chair yoga. Meet Sarah, a resilient individual whose life took an unexpected turn when she was diagnosed with multiple sclerosis. Amid the uncertainty enveloped her, Sarah discovered an unexpected ally in the form of a simple chair.

Sarah's journey was marked by the daily challenges posed by her neurological condition. The once-fluid movements of her body were replaced by stiffness and discomfort. Everyday tasks became hurdles, and the fear of falling loomed large. Amid this adversity, Sarah encountered chair yoga—a practice that would become her anchor in the storm.

At first, the idea of yoga seemed daunting, considering her physical limitations. However, introducing a chair into the practice proved to be a game-changer. With gentle guidance, Sarah learned to synchronize her breath with purposeful movements, all from the supportive seat of her chair.

As days turned into weeks and weeks into months, Sarah's journey with chair yoga unfolded like the petals of a resilient flower. The once-stiff joints began to regain mobility, and the fear of falls gradually dissipated. Once a symbol of rest, the chair became a vessel of empowerment, carrying Sarah through a journey of self-discovery and healing.

Through consistent and mindful engagement with chair yoga, Sarah experienced physical improvement and a profound shift in her mental and emotional well-being. Sitting and moving mindfully became a sanctuary where she found solace, strength, and a renewed sense of agency in her health.

Sarah's story is not an isolated incident but a testament to the universal potential embedded in chair yoga. It is a narrative that echoes the transformative possibilities of approaching mindful movement with an open heart and a chair as a supportive companion.

As we delve into the heart of "Mindful Movement," let Sarah's journey be a beacon—a living testament to the remarkable changes that can unfold when one embraces the simplicity and accessibility of chair yoga.

"Mindful Movement: Chair Yoga for Neurological Well-being" is a comprehensive guide tailored to address your specific needs as an individual with a neurological condition, such as multiple sclerosis, Parkinson's disease, or fibromyalgia. This book offers accessible and effective chair yoga routines designed to help you overcome the challenges and limitations posed by your condition.

Living with a neurological condition can present physical, emotional, and mental obstacles that significantly impact your quality of life. Symptoms like muscle weakness, tremors, fatigue, pain, and limited mobility can make traditional physical activities difficult. This book aims to fill the need for specialized wellness practices that cater to these challenges and promote your overall well-being.

The mission is to provide you with chair yoga routines specifically adapted to your needs. These routines are carefully crafted to promote flexibility, strength, balance, and relaxation while considering the unique challenges of your condition. The book also emphasizes the importance of mindfulness in movement, helping you develop a deeper connection with your body, manage stress and anxiety, and enhance your overall well-being.

Individuals living with neurological conditions often encounter physical challenges such as muscle weakness and limited mobility, emotional challenges like stress and anxiety, and mental challenges that can impact their overall well-being. Due to these challenges, traditional forms of physical activity may be difficult to engage in. As a result, there is a growing need for specialized wellness practices that can accommodate these obstacles and promote overall well-being.

The chair yoga routines presented in this book are carefully designed to address the diverse needs of individuals with neurological conditions. Each routine is tailored to promote flexibility, strength, balance, and relaxation while considering the specific challenges posed by each condition. Clear and easy-to-follow instructions, accompanied by illustrations and modifications, are provided to make yoga accessible to individuals with varying abilities and limitations.

Moreover, the book emphasizes the importance of mindfulness in movement, encouraging individuals to cultivate a deeper awareness of their bodies and breath. Mindful movement practices can help individuals with neurological conditions develop a greater sense of connection with their bodies, manage stress and anxiety, and enhance their overall well-being. This book provides a comprehensive approach to well-being that tackles the mental, emotional, and physical elements of living with a neurological illness by incorporating mindfulness into chair yoga exercises.

Chair Yoga for Neurological Well-being" empowers you to enhance your quality of life and well-being through accessible and effective chair yoga routines tailored to your neurological condition. With a focus on mindful movement and a comprehensive approach to well-being, the book will help you overcome your condition's obstacles and improve your quality of life in general.

The book's central subject is a potent and comprehensive strategy for meeting the requirements of people with neurological illnesses is to "Empower individuals with neurological conditions through mindful movement for improved weight management, pain relief, balance, and strength." This theme emphasizes the transformative potential of mindful movement practices, such as chair yoga, in enhancing various aspects of well-being for individuals facing neurological challenges. You may enhance your ability to control your weight, discomfort, balance, strength, and overall well-being by adding mindful movement into your daily routine. This will ultimately give you the confidence to take charge of your health and well-being.

A neurological disorder can cause a variety of mental, emotional, and physical difficulties that can seriously lower your quality of life. Symptoms such as muscle weakness, tremors, fatigue, pain, and limited mobility can make traditional physical activity difficult. This can lead to challenges in weight management, as well as increased discomfort and reduced mobility due to pain and muscle stiffness. Maintaining balance and strength can also become more challenging, impacting your overall physical well-being.

The main theme underscores the idea that mindful movement practices can be a transformative tool for individuals with neurological conditions. By engaging in mindful movements, such as chair yoga, you can actively address these challenges and work towards improving your overall well-being.

Mindful movement practices, such as chair yoga, can improve weight management by promoting physical activity and enhancing body awareness. Regular mindful movement routines can help you maintain a healthy weight by supporting metabolism and promoting well-being. Additionally, mindful movement can foster a positive relationship with your body, encouraging mindful eating and healthy lifestyle choices to contribute to weight management.

It is well established that mindful movement techniques can help those with chronic pain. Incorporating gentle and intentional movements into your daily routine can alleviate muscle tension, reduce discomfort, and improve your overall sense of physical comfort. Mindful movement can also help you develop a greater awareness of your body's signals, allowing you to respond to pain proactively and empoweringly.

Individuals with neurological conditions may experience challenges related to balance and coordination. Mindful movement practices, such as chair yoga, can help improve balance by focusing on stability, posture, and controlled movements. Regular practice can enhance your proprioception and spatial awareness, leading to improved balance and a reduced risk of falls or accidents.

Maintaining physical strength is essential for individuals with neurological conditions, as it can support mobility and overall well-being. Mindful movement practices, including chair yoga, promote strength through gentle yet effective movements. You may steadily increase and preserve your muscle strength by doing these exercises, which will help you carry out everyday tasks more confidently and easily.

The main theme emphasizes the empowerment of individuals with neurological conditions through mindful movement. You can actively manage your health and well-being by incorporating these practices into your daily routine. The mindful movement offers a holistic approach that addresses the physical aspects of your condition and the emotional and mental dimensions of your well-being.

This theme in mind is a guiding principle for integrating mindful movement practices into your life. By embracing this theme, you can journey towards improved well-being, enhanced physical comfort, and greater empowerment in managing the challenges associated with your neurological condition.

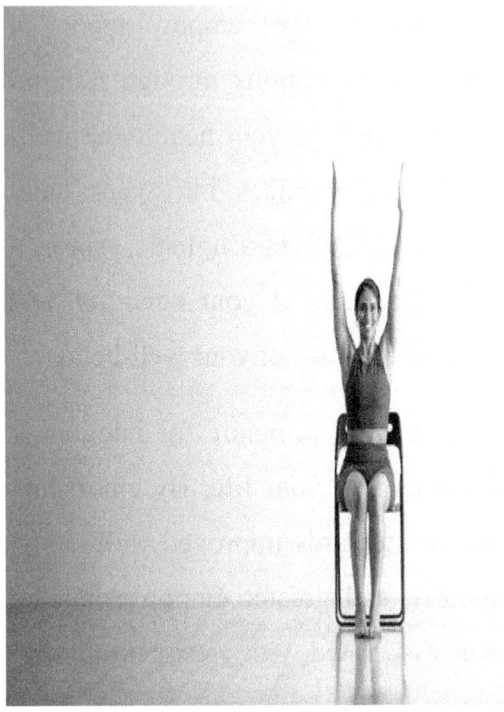

CHAPTER 1

Understanding Chair Yoga for Neurological Well-being

As we embark on this journey of understanding chair yoga for neurological well-being, we must begin with a startling fact about the prevalence of neurological conditions. Millions of individuals worldwide suffer from neurological illnesses, the most frequent of which are multiple sclerosis, Parkinson's disease, and fibromyalgia, according to the World Health Organisation. These illnesses can have a substantial influence on a person's life and offer a variety of physical, emotional, and mental difficulties that need specific care and attention.

Neurological conditions are more prevalent than many people realize, with millions of individuals facing the daily realities of these disorders. The impact of these conditions extends beyond the individuals themselves, affecting their families, caregivers, and communities. Understanding the widespread prevalence of neurological conditions is crucial in recognizing the urgent need for effective and accessible wellness practices tailored to address the unique challenges those living with these conditions face.

By shedding light on the prevalence of neurological disorders, we can appreciate the significance of developing specialized approaches to support individuals in managing their well-being. This understanding underscores the importance of exploring chair yoga as a valuable tool for promoting neurological well-being. Chair yoga is a gentle and flexible mindful movement practice that may be customized to meet the requirements and physical constraints of people with neurological problems.

As we delve deeper into the exploration of chair yoga for neurological well-being, it becomes clear that this practice holds the potential to empower individuals to engage in their care actively. By understanding the prevalence of neurological conditions and their challenges, we can approach the practice of chair yoga with a sense of purpose and urgency, recognizing its capacity to impact the lives of those affected by these conditions positively.

In the following chapters, we will further explore the principles and techniques of chair yoga, examining how this practice can address the physical, emotional, and mental aspects of living with a neurological condition. By gaining a thorough awareness of chair yoga and its possible advantages, we can arm ourselves with the information and resources to set a path toward enhanced well-being and more self-determination.

Neurological Conditions and the Body-Mind Connection

As we continue our exploration, it's important to remember the individuals whose lives are touched by neurological conditions. By acknowledging the prevalence of these disorders and their impact on countless lives, we can approach the study of chair yoga for neurological well-being with a deep sense of empathy and purpose. Our journey begins with this understanding, laying the foundation for a meaningful and impactful exploration of chair yoga as a pathway to improved well-being for individuals facing neurological challenges.

Living with a neurological condition can present various challenges in your daily life. These challenges can affect you physically, emotionally, and mentally. However, chair yoga can offer significant benefits that address these different aspects of your well-being.

Let's start with the physical aspect. Chair yoga is about finding gentle ways to move and stretch your body, even when faced with physical limitations. It can help improve flexibility, build strength, enhance balance, and promote relaxation. These physical benefits are crucial for individuals with neurological conditions, as they can help you manage symptoms such as muscle weakness, stiffness, and limited mobility. By engaging in chair yoga, you can work towards maintaining and improving your physical abilities, which is essential for your overall well-being.

Chair yoga offers a gentle yet effective way for individuals with neurological conditions to improve their physical well-being. Even though diseases like multiple sclerosis, Parkinson's disease, or stroke might be difficult to manage, chair yoga can help with general physical ability and symptom management. In this thorough investigation, we will focus on the particular physical advantages of chair yoga for people with neurological disorders, highlighting its capacity to increase strength, flexibility, balance, and relaxation. By understanding the profound impact of chair yoga on physical well-being, we can establish its significance as a valuable tool for managing symptoms and improving overall quality of life.

Flexibility is a key component of physical well-being, particularly for individuals with neurological conditions. A simple, accessible method of increasing flexibility via light stretching and exercise is chair yoga. The method's main goal is to progressively increase the joint range of motion, easing muscle stiffness and lowering the chance of contractures. By engaging in regular chair yoga routines, individuals can experience improved flexibility, making daily movements and activities more comfortable and manageable.

Furthermore, building strength is essential for individuals facing neurological challenges. Chair yoga incorporates various strength-building exercises that target different muscle groups. These exercises are adapted to be performed while seated, allowing you to engage in strength training without putting excessive strain on their bodies. By consistently practicing chair yoga, individuals can strengthen their muscles, contributing to better posture, enhanced stability, and improved overall physical function.

Enhancing balance is another critical aspect of physical well-being, especially for you with neurological conditions that may affect coordination and stability. Chair yoga includes specific poses and movements designed to promote balance and proprioception. By engaging in these activities that enhance balance, you can become more stable and lower their chance of falling or getting into an accident. Enhanced balance can significantly impact daily activities, leading to greater confidence and independence in movement.

Moreover, promoting relaxation is an integral part of chair yoga practice. Incorporating breathing techniques, mindfulness, and gentle movements in char yoga routines creates a relaxing environment. Individuals with neurological conditions often experience heightened stress and tension, which can exacerbate symptoms and impact overall well-being. Through chair yoga, you can learn to release physical and mental tension, promoting a sense of calm and relaxation.

This relaxation response can positively impact the nervous system, potentially reducing the intensity of symptoms and improving overall comfort. By engaging in chair yoga, individuals with neurological conditions can work towards maintaining and improving their physical abilities, which is essential for their overall well-being. The gentle and adaptable nature of chair yoga makes it suitable for you with varying mobility and physical capabilities. It offers a safe space for people to move and work out, encouraging self-determination and well-being.

Now, let's talk about the emotional impact. Managing a neurological illness can be an emotional rollercoaster. Tensions, anxieties, and annoyances might be part of the daily script. But here's the silver lining – chair yoga steps in as your emotional anchor. It's not just about poses; it's about forging a deeper connection between you and your emotions, creating a haven where you can find peace amidst the emotional whirlwind.

Living with a neurological illness isn't just a physical challenge; it's an emotional one, too. It's like carrying an invisible backpack filled with uncertainties, frustrations, and moments of self-doubt.

Tensions can bubble up, anxieties might linger, and annoyance can become a familiar companion. It's a lot to carry, and let's be honest, it takes a toll on the emotional landscape.

Enter chair yoga – not just as a set of physical exercises but as a technique to wrangle those emotions. It's like a toolbox for your feelings, offering a way to navigate the emotional waves that come with the territory of a neurological condition. How does it work? Well, let's break it down.

- **Deeper Connection:**

Chair yoga acts as a bridge between your body and your emotions. It's not just about the physical postures; it's a journey inward. The chair becomes more than just a prop; it's a companion in this exploration of your emotional landscape. Each movement, each breath becomes a conversation with your emotions, an acknowledgment of what you're feeling in that moment.

Imagine a simple stretch – it's not just about reaching out physically; it becomes a gesture of reaching inwards, connecting with the emotions lingering beneath the surface. The chair supports you and becomes a stable base for this exploration, creating a safe space to unravel the complexities of your emotional world.

- **Mindfulness in Motion:**

Now, let's talk mindfulness. Chair yoga is like a gentle guide into the realm of mindfulness. It encourages you to be present – not just physically present but emotionally, too. As you move through the poses, it's an invitation to be aware of your thoughts and feelings without judgment. It's about creating a conscious connection between your body and your emotional state.

Mindfulness in motion means acknowledging that there might be tension, anxiety, or annoyance, and that's okay. It's not about pushing these feelings away but inviting them into the conversation. The chair becomes your anchor in this mindful voyage, grounding you in the present moment and fostering a deeper understanding of your emotional landscape.

- **Cultivating Calm and Inner Peace:**

Now, the magic happens. As you breathe through the movements and become mindful of each stretch, there's a gradual cultivation of calm and inner peace. It's not a quick fix; it's a gradual unfolding. Chair yoga becomes a toolkit for emotional resilience, offering a space to process, accept, and release.

The intentional breathing, synchronized with purposeful movements, becomes a balm for the emotional turbulence. It's a practice that says, " let's take a moment to acknowledge what you're feeling, and then let's release what doesn't serve you." In this process, the chair transforms into a sanctuary, a haven where you can release some of the emotional burdens you've been carrying.

- **Breathing Room for Your Emotions:**

Picture chair yoga as creating breathing room for your emotions. In each pose, with every inhale and exhale, there's space for your feelings to exist without overwhelming you. It's like letting fresh air and clarity flood a stuffy room when you open a window.

Chair yoga provides a similar breathing room for your emotions, allowing you to acknowledge them without being suffocated by their weight.

Here's the beautiful part – chair yoga becomes a haven for emotional release. As you flow through the movements and surrender into each pose, there's an opportunity to let go. It's not about denying or suppressing; it's about acknowledging, expressing, and gently releasing.

Think of it like this – you might be holding onto stress, worry, or frustration. Chair yoga invites you to consciously exhale these emotions, to release them with each breath. The chair stands as a witness, a support in this process of emotional unburdening. It's a sacred space where you can shed some of the emotional weight that comes with the territory of neurological challenges.

Chair yoga isn't just a series of movements; it's your emotional retreat. It's a practice that invites you to explore the intricate dance between your body and your emotions. Through mindfulness, intentional breathing, and the support of a chair, it becomes a sanctuary where you can find calm amidst the storm of emotions.

So, as you engage in chair yoga, see it as a journey to forge a deeper connection with your emotions, cultivate a sense of peace within, and create a breathing room where your feelings can exist without overwhelming you. It's not a cure for the emotional challenges of a neurological condition, but it's a powerful tool. In this haven, you can find solace amid emotional complexity.

Finally, let's consider the mental aspect. Living with a neurological condition can, sometimes, feel overwhelming, and it's important to take care of your mental well-being. Chair yoga can help you clear your mind, improve your focus, and build mental resilience. By engaging in the practice, you can cultivate a positive mindset and feel more in control of your thoughts and emotions. Living with a neurological disease comes with ups and downs, and this mental clarity and sense of empowerment are crucial for managing them.

By understanding how chair yoga can positively impact you physically, emotionally, and mentally, we can establish the foundation for its connection to your overall well-being. It's not just about exercise; it's about finding a holistic approach to support your journey. Chair yoga offers a way to address your multifaceted challenges and promote a sense of well-being that encompasses your entire being.

In conclusion, chair yoga has the potential to make a real difference in your life. It's about finding gentle movement, emotional support, and mental clarity. By recognizing the holistic benefits of chair yoga, we can lay the groundwork for a meaningful and impactful exploration of this practice as a pathway to improved well-being for you as you face the challenges of living with a neurological condition.

In summary, chair yoga offers a holistic approach to well-being for individuals with neurological conditions. It addresses these conditions' physical, emotional, and mental challenges, providing a comprehensive framework for improving overall quality of life. Chair yoga can be useful for people with neurological problems to manage symptoms, reduce stress, and promote well-being via moderate movement, awareness, and empowerment.

The physical benefits of chair yoga are particularly significant for individuals with neurological conditions.

The gentle movements and stretches can help improve flexibility, build strength, enhance balance, and promote relaxation. These physical improvements can directly address symptoms such as muscle weakness, stiffness, and limited mobility, ultimately contributing to an improved quality of life.

Emotionally, chair yoga can provide a supportive space for individuals to connect with their bodies and cultivate mindfulness. This can lead to a greater sense of calm and inner peace, helping individuals manage the emotional challenges often accompanying neurological conditions. Chair yoga can offer emotional relief and support by creating a space for relaxation and self-awareness.

Mentally, chair yoga can help individuals clear their minds, improve focus, and build resilience. The practice encourages a positive mindset and a sense of empowerment, providing individuals with tools to navigate the mental challenges associated with neurological conditions. By promoting mental clarity and a feeling of control, chair yoga can contribute to a more balanced and resilient approach to daily life.

Chair yoga creates a comprehensive framework for addressing the many obstacles of living with a neurological illness by acknowledging the interdependence of physical, emotional, and mental well-being. It provides a thorough method for raising people's general quality of life and gives them the tools to take an active role in their care and well-being.

Benefits of Mindful Movement

Through gentle movement, mindfulness, and empowerment, chair yoga becomes a powerful tool for managing symptoms, reducing stress, and promoting well-being in the face of neurological challenges. Lets examine some of the benefits of this Mindful practice:

1. Mindful Movement for the Win:

Chair yoga isn't just about random stretches; it's like a mindful dance for your nerves. When you move, especially with the support of a chair, it sends signals to your brain. These signals create a roadmap for your nerves, reminding them to communicate and coordinate better. It's like giving your nervous system a friendly nudge in the right direction.

2. Breathing the Good Vibes:

Chair yoga pairs movements with intentional breathing. It's not just about inhaling and exhaling; it's about giving your brain and nerves a steady supply of oxygen. Imagine it as a breath of fresh air for your whole system. This oxygen boost tells your nerves, " we're in this together, let's stay calm and collected."

3. Stress-Buster Extraordinaire:

Stress is like the villain in this story of neurological challenges. Chair yoga steps in as the hero, armed with relaxation techniques. When you're stressed, your body reacts, and it's not always friendly to your nerves. Chair yoga introduces moves that tell your muscles to chill out. As your muscles relax, it sends a message to your nerves – "All is well, no need to sound the alarms." It's like a superhero saving the day but in a chair.

4. Balancing Act for Your Brain:

Do you know that feeling when your balance is a bit wonky? Chair yoga is like your secret weapon for finding your center. The movements, even those done sitting down, work on your stability. It's not about doing circus acts; it's about creating a solid foundation for your brain to trust. When your brain feels secure, it sends signals that help your overall coordination and balance.

5. Strength Training, Chair-Style:

Chair yoga isn't about bench-pressing but gradual, gentle strength-building. As you move through the poses, your muscles get a workout. Stronger muscles mean better support for your nerves. It's like giving your nerves a team of bodyguards – they feel safer and more secure in their surroundings. Plus, it's a bonus for your overall physical well-being.

6. Happy Chemicals on the Move:

Here's a cool science bit – when you move, your brain releases these awesome chemicals called endorphins. They're like the happy messengers in your body. Chair yoga, even in its seated glory, encourages the release of these endorphins. So, while making these moves, you're not just physically helping your nerves but also giving your mood a little lift.

7. Your Personal Timeout Space:

Lastly, chair yoga is your timeout amid the chaos. Life with neurological challenges can be overwhelming. Chair yoga creates a little bubble where you can breathe, move, and let go of some of the weight you're carrying. This mental break is crucial. It's not just about the poses; it's about creating a positive atmosphere.

Testimony: Meet Sarah, a spirited woman in her mid-50s whose journey with neurological challenges took an unexpected turn toward relief through the gentle practice of chair yoga.

Sarah had been living with multiple sclerosis (MS) for over a decade, a condition that brought its share of physical and emotional trials. The unpredictability of MS had woven a tapestry of uncertainties into Sarah's daily life. Fatigue, muscle weakness, and balance issues became uninvited companions on her journey.

As the years passed, Sarah gradually surrendered to the limitations imposed by her condition. Everyday activities became more daunting, and the fear of falling overshadowed her once-vibrant spirit. Traditional exercise routines seemed like an unattainable goal, and searching for a practice that could offer solace and physical engagement led her to chair yoga.

Enter Claire, a seasoned chair yoga instructor with a compassionate approach. Claire understood the nuances of adapting yoga for those with neurological conditions, recognizing the unique challenges individuals like Sarah's face. Their first meeting unfolded in a cozy community center, where a circle of chairs awaited a group eager to explore the benefits of mindful movement.

For Sarah, the initial sessions were more than just physical exercises; they were a lifeline. The chair became her anchor, providing security as she navigated through gentle stretches and breathing exercises. Claire's guidance encouraged Sarah to listen to her body, honoring its signals without judgment.

The first notable shift came in the realm of pain relief. Accustomed to the persistent muscle ache, Sarah experienced moments of respite after each chair yoga session. The carefully crafted movements and focused breathing coaxed her body into a state of relaxation that transcended the physical realm.

As the weeks passed, Sarah noticed improved balance, a facet of her life that had been steadily eroding. Seated poses like the modified tree pose became a source of empowerment. The chair provided a stabilizing force, allowing Sarah to concentrate on the subtleties of her body's movements without fearing losing balance.

Perhaps the most profound transformation occurred in Sarah's mental well-being. The rhythm of chair yoga became a meditation in motion, a respite from the daily concerns that often crowded her mind. With each session, a sense of mindfulness settled in, creating a mental sanctuary where worries momentarily faded.

One pivotal day, Sarah rose from her chair with an ease she hadn't felt in years. The once arduous movements became more fluid, and a newfound strength seemed to emanate from the core of her being. It wasn't a miraculous cure, but it was a testament to the resilience of the human spirit when nurtured with care and intention.

The community that formed within the chair yoga group became a source of support and camaraderie. Sarah's journey became intertwined with fellow participants, each contributing to the shared tapestry of encouragement and understanding.

While chair yoga didn't erase the challenges posed by MS, it became a transformative force in Sarah's life. It was a practice that embraced her limitations, celebrated her progress, and, most importantly, offered a sense of agency over her well-being. Sarah's story is a testament to the healing potential embedded in the mindful movements of chair yoga, proving that relief can emerge from unexpected places, even from the simple act of sitting in a chair and moving with intention.

So, there you have it – chair yoga is like a superhero, a mood booster, and a nerve-friendly workout all rolled into one. Your body says, "Thanks for the love; I needed that." So, grab a chair, sit, and give your nerves a little TLC with chair yoga magic!

CHAPTER 2

Weight Management through Mindful Movement

You know, our bodies are pretty complex, and when it comes to neurological conditions, they can add an extra layer of complexity, especially in the weight department.

How Neurological Conditions Can Affect Weight

1. Disrupted Signals Between Brain and Body:

Neurological conditions disrupt the intricate communication network between the brain and the rest of the body. This communication is vital for regulating various physiological functions, including weight-related ones. When these signals go awry, the body receives mixed messages, impacting how it processes and responds to food, energy, and movement.

2. Altered Appetite and Metabolism:

The disruptions caused by neurological conditions can manifest in changes to appetite and metabolism. For some individuals, there might be a decrease in appetite, leading to unintended weight loss. Others may experience an increase in appetite or changes in metabolism, making weight management a more nuanced challenge. The body's usual regulatory mechanisms for energy intake and expenditure become irregular.

3. Impact on Mobility:

The impact on mobility is one important factor. People who have multiple sclerosis or Parkinson's disease may find it more difficult to exercise since these illnesses might affect motor function. If eating choices don't alter, decreased mobility can lower daily energy expenditure and result in weight gain. It becomes a delicate balance between managing mobility limitations and maintaining an active lifestyle.

4. Energy Levels and Fatigue:

Neurological conditions often come with the unwelcome companion of fatigue. Feeling constantly tired can hinder the motivation to engage in physical activities. This fatigue can create a cycle where decreased energy levels contribute to reduced physical activity, further impacting weight management.

5. Medication Side Effects:

Many individuals with neurological conditions rely on medications to manage symptoms. However, these medications may come with side effects that directly influence weight. Some medications can alter appetite, leading to increased or decreased food intake. Additionally, certain medications might cause fluid retention or metabolic changes, contributing to fluctuations in weight.

6. Emotional and Psychological Factors:

Living with a neurological condition can bring about emotional and psychological challenges. Stress, anxiety, or depression, which are common companions to these conditions, can influence eating habits. Some individuals may turn to food for comfort, while others may experience a loss of appetite due to emotional distress.

7. Individual Variability:

Recognizing the individual variability in how neurological conditions impact weight is essential. Each person's experience is unique, and factors such as the specific type of neurological condition, its severity, and the presence of other health conditions contribute to the overall picture.

Navigating weight management in the context of neurological conditions is indeed like solving a puzzle. It requires a comprehensive and individualized approach that addresses each person's specific challenges. This could involve a combination of adaptive physical activity, mindful eating practices, and close monitoring of medication effects, all under the guidance of healthcare professionals specializing in neurological care.

The Role of Chair Yoga in Creating a Foundation for Weight Management

Now, let's talk about chair yoga—a game-changer for creating a foundation for weight management, especially in these neurological challenges.

1. Adaptability and Accessibility:

Here's the beauty of chair yoga—it's like a fitness buddy that meets you where you are. The chair provides support, making it accessible for individuals with various mobility levels. Whether you're dealing with limited mobility or fatigue, chair yoga has your back (or, should I say, your seat).

2. Mindful Movement and Weight Management:

Chair yoga is not just about physical exercise but mindful movement. Those gentle stretches and intentional poses connect your body and mind. It's like a dance that encourages awareness of how your body moves and feels.

This mindfulness aspect is gold for weight management. Being present now makes you more alert to your body's signals, including hunger and fullness. It's like chair yoga, laying the foundation for a more mindful approach to eating and moving.

3. Building Strength and Burning Calories:

Those simple movements can engage various muscle groups, contributing to overall strength. Plus, the energy expended in these mindful movements adds up, helping with calorie burning—the good old equation for weight management.

4. Stress Reduction and Emotional Well-being:

Here's a kicker—chair yoga is not just about the physical stuff. It's also a stress-buster. Managing stress is crucial for weight management because stress can affect our eating habits. Chair yoga's calming effect can positively impact emotional well-being, making it a holistic tool for weight management.

Chair Yoga Routines for Calorie Burn

1. Seated Marching:

- Sit comfortably on the chair with your feet flat on the ground and your back straight.
- Lift your right knee towards your chest, mimicking a marching motion.
- To increase the intensity of your lift, contract your core muscles.
- Lower your right foot and repeat with the left knee.
- Gradually increase the pace, keeping the movement controlled.

- Aim for a rhythmic motion, lifting and lowering each knee.

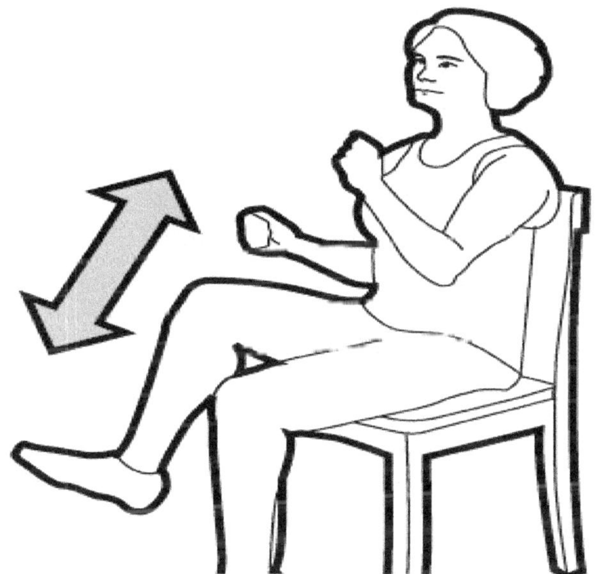

2. Seated Jumping Jacks:

- Stay seated with your back straight and legs together.
- Open your legs to the sides while simultaneously raising your arms overhead.
- Return to the starting position by bringing your legs together and lowering your arms.
- Keep the movement controlled to avoid strain.

- This low-impact version of jumping jacks elevates your heart rate without stressing your joints.

Seated Jumping Jacks

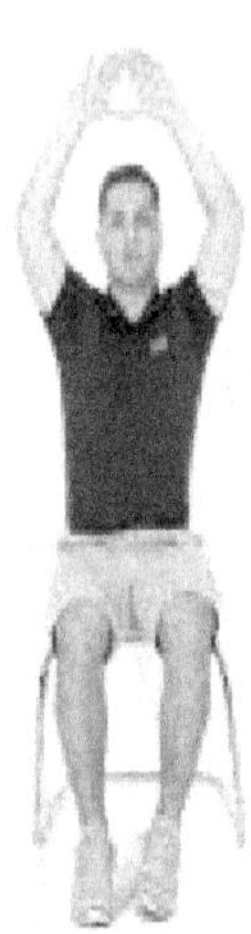

3. Seated Side Taps:

- Sit at the edge of the chair, maintaining good posture.
- Tap your right foot to the side, then return it to the center.
- Repeat the same motion with your left foot.
- Add an arms reach towards the side you're tapping to intensify the movement.

- This targets your thighs, hips, and obliques, contributing to calorie burn.

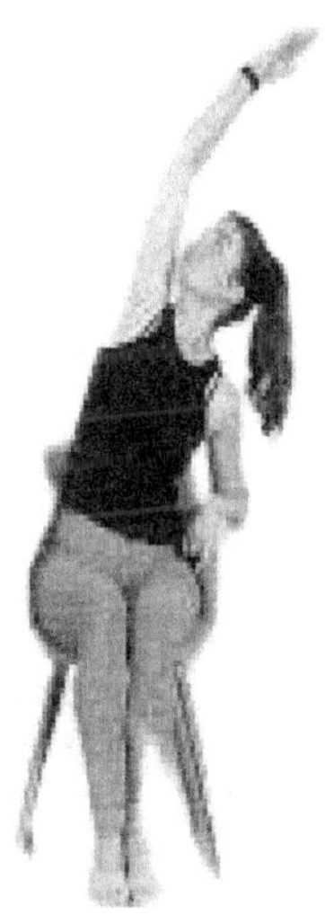

4. Seated Twist and Reach:

- Sit tall with your spine straight and feet flat on the floor.
- Inhale and exhale as you twist your torso to the right and reach your left hand towards the back of the chair.
- Inhale back to the center and repeat on the other side.

- Engage your core during the twist to work those abdominal muscles.
- This movement not only burns calories but also promotes flexibility in your spine.

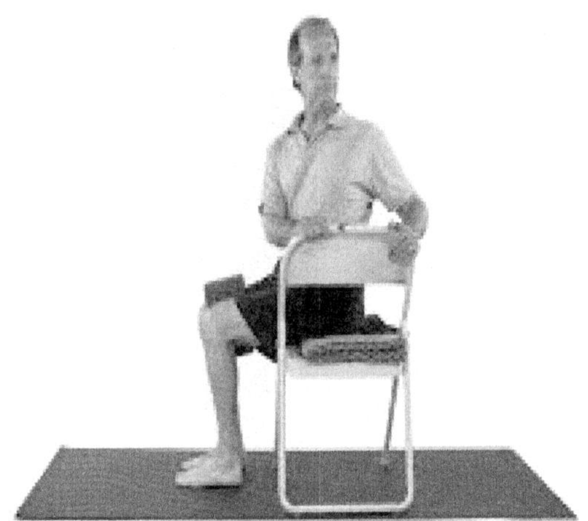

5. Arm Circles:

- Raise your arms shoulder height to the sides.
- Start with tiny circles and move your arms in circles.
- Make little circular movements with your arms at first.
- This engages your shoulder and arm muscles.

- Continue the circular motion for a set duration, ensuring controlled and deliberate movements.

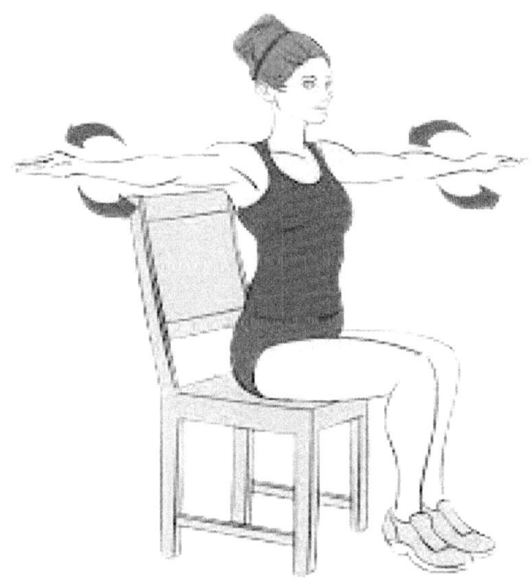

Remember, the key to effective calorie burn with Chair Yoga is maintaining control, engaging your core, and gradually increasing the intensity.

These routines are designed to be gentle yet effective, making them accessible for various fitness levels. Listen to your body and modify the movements to suit your comfort and ability.

Incorporating Mindful Eating Practices

Now, let's talk about mindful eating because it goes hand in hand with your Chair Yoga routines for a holistic approach to well-being.

1. Mindful Awareness:

Before you eat, take a moment to check in with your body. Are you hungry, or is it more of an emotional or habitual craving? This awareness sets the stage for mindful eating.

2. Savor Each Bite:

As you eat, savor each bite. Pay attention to the flavors, textures, and sensations. This enhances your eating experience and allows your brain to register satisfaction more effectively.

3. Slow Down:

During meals, pace yourself. Please slow down and allow your body to recognize when it's full. Savouring your meal slowly might help you avoid overeating since it takes some time for signals from your stomach to reach your brain.

4. Listen to Your Body:

Pay attention to your body's cues of hunger and fullness. Stop eating when you feel satisfied, even if there's still food on your plate. It's about honoring your body's signals.

5. Eliminate Distractions:

Turn off the TV, put away your phone, and create a calm eating environment. Removing distractions helps you stay present and focused on your meal, fostering a more mindful eating experience.

6. Portion Control:

Be mindful of portion sizes. Use smaller plates to help regulate the amount of food you serve yourself. It's a simple yet effective strategy for maintaining a healthy balance.

By combining Chair Yoga routines for calorie burn with mindful eating practices, you're not just exercising your body but cultivating a holistic approach to health. It's a dynamic duo supporting your physical and mental well-being, promoting a balanced and sustainable lifestyle.

Let's talk about building a sustainable weight management routine involving a tailored chair yoga practice. We'll take this journey together, focusing on creating a routine that suits your goals and emphasizing the importance of consistency and mindfulness.

What specific weight management goals do you have? Knowing your goals—losing weight, keeping it off, or feeling better overall—will help you create a programme that works for you.

Designing Your Chair Yoga Routine

Tailoring a chair yoga routine for weight management involves selecting movements that engage various muscle groups, elevate the heart rate, and promote flexibility. Here's a simple guide to get you started:

a. Seated Marching: Lift your knees individually, engaging your core. Gradually increase the pace.

b. Seated Jumping Jacks: Open and close your legs and arms in a controlled motion.

c. Seated Side Taps: Tap one foot to the side, incorporating an arm reach for intensity.

d. Seated Twist and Reach: Twist your torso, reaching towards the back of the chair, engaging your core.

e. Arm Circles: Extend your arms and make circular motions, gradually increasing the size.

Consistency is Key

Now, let's talk about consistency. It's the secret sauce in any successful routine. Aim for regularity rather than intensity. Start with a realistic schedule, a few times a week, and gradually build up. Consistency breeds habit, and habits lead to lasting change. Mindfulness is the anchor that keeps your routine sustainable.

During your chair yoga practice:

a. Focus on Your Breath: Connect your movements with your breath. Inhale during stretches exhale during contractions.

b. Be Present: Pay attention to how your body feels during each movement. Mindful awareness enhances the effectiveness of your routine.

c. Appreciate Progress: Celebrate small victories. Acknowledge the positive changes, whether it's increased flexibility or a boost in energy.

Weight management is a journey, not a sprint. As you become comfortable with your chair yoga routine, consider making gradual progressions. This might involve adding more repetitions, increasing the duration, or exploring additional movements. Your body is your guide. If a particular movement feels challenging, that's okay. Adapt it to your comfort level. The goal is to enjoy the process, not to strain yourself.

Periodically reflect on your routine. How does it make you feel? Are you noticing any changes in your body or energy levels? Based on your observations, make adjustments to keep the routine engaging and aligned with your evolving goals.

Testimony: Lets revisit the story of Sarah like we stated before, a vibrant individual navigating the challenges of weight management while dealing with chronic pain due to fibromyalgia. Sarah's journey began when she explored alternative approaches to support her well-being. Traditional workouts were often too strenuous, exacerbating her pain, and the idea of chair yoga caught her attention.

Sarah started with simple chair yoga routines tailored to her needs. Seated marches, gentle twists, and arm circles became her companions in this new fitness venture. The support of the chair provided stability, allowing her to engage in effective and pain-free movements. Consistency became Sarah's mantra. She started with short sessions several times a week, gradually increasing the duration as her confidence and comfort grew.

The beauty of chair yoga, she found, was in its adaptability. Even when the pain was more challenging, Sarah could modify her routine without compromising the essence of the practice. Simultaneously, Sarah began incorporating mindful eating practices into her daily routine. Being present during meals, savouring each bite, and recognizing hunger and fullness cues became integral to her lifestyle.

The synergy of chair yoga and mindful eating created a holistic approach to weight management that felt sustainable. Over time, Sarah noticed a transformation. The pounds started to shed gradually, but more importantly, she felt renewed energy and well-being. Chair yoga provided a means for calorie burn and became a source of emotional support. The mindfulness cultivated during her practice extended beyond the mat, influencing her relationship with food and her body.

Sarah's journey sheds light on the interconnected nature of pain and weight management. Here's how:

1. Physical Activity and Pain Relief:

With its gentle yet effective movements, chair yoga became a tool for pain relief. Engaging in regular physical activity helped alleviate the stiffness associated with fibromyalgia.

As pain decreased, Sarah became more motivated to move, creating a positive cycle.

2. Mind-Body Connection:

The mindfulness fostered during chair yoga extended to pain management. Sarah learned to listen to her body's signals, distinguishing between discomfort and pain. This awareness empowered her to make choices that supported both her weight and pain management goals.

3. Emotional Well-being:

Chronic pain can affect emotional well-being, often leading to emotional eating. Chair yoga, emphasizing mindfulness, provided a coping mechanism for stress and emotional challenges. As their emotional well-being improved, Sarah was less inclined to turn to food for comfort.

4. Improved Sleep:

Many individuals dealing with chronic pain face sleep disturbances. Chair yoga's calming effects positively influenced Sarah's sleep patterns. Improved sleep, in turn, contributed to better weight management by regulating hormonal balance related to appetite.

In Sarah's story, chair yoga became a catalyst for holistic well-being, demonstrating that weight and pain management are not isolated endeavours but interconnected aspects of a person's health journey. This narrative emphasizes the transformative power of a mindful and adaptive approach to fitness and lifestyle.

CHAPTER 3

Pain Management Practices for Neurological Well-being

Neurological pain, a complex symphony of sensations, often accompanies conditions such as multiple sclerosis (MS), Parkinson's disease, and fibromyalgia. Delving into the intricacies of these conditions sheds light on the diverse types of pain individuals may experience and their profound impact on their overall well-being.

Types of Pain Associated with Fibromyalgia

Fibromyalgia, a chronic disorder with a multifaceted impact on the body, mind, and daily life, is characterized by widespread musculoskeletal pain, tenderness, and fatigue. While the exact cause remains elusive, the condition is associated with alterations in how the nervous system processes pain signals, leading to heightened sensitivity and discomfort.

Pains associated with Fibromyagia include:

- **Widespread Muscular Pain:**

Fibromyalgia is renowned for its hallmark symptom—widespread muscular pain. Many people describe this pain as a persistent, dull discomfort that affects several bodily components, such as tendons, ligaments, and muscles.

- **Hyperalgesia and Allodynia:**

Hyperalgesia, or increased sensitivity to pain, and allodynia, or discomfort from stimuli that are normally painless, are two possible symptoms of fibromyalgia.

Everyday activities, such as being touched or lightly bumped, can become sources of discomfort.

- **Joint Pain:**

Joint pain is another facet of fibromyalgia, contributing to stiffness and soreness. This pain can affect small and large joints and is often exacerbated by physical activity.

The Impact of Pain on Overall Well-being

Regardless of its specific manifestation, neurological pain casts a wide-reaching shadow on overall well-being. Its impact extends beyond the physical realm, seeping into emotional and mental dimensions.

1. Emotional Toll:

Chronic pain, a constant companion for many with neurological conditions, can contribute to heightened stress, anxiety, and depression. The persistent nature of pain becomes an emotional burden, impacting one's quality of life.

2. Disruption of Sleep:

Neurological pain often disrupts sleep patterns, leading to fatigue and exacerbating other symptoms associated with the underlying conditions. It might be difficult to stop the cycle of pain and sleep disruption that they generate together.

3. Limitation of Daily Activities:

Pain can significantly curtail daily activities, affecting mobility, independence, and the ability to engage in social and recreational pursuits. The limitations imposed by pain contribute to a sense of loss and frustration.

4. Cognitive Impacts:

Neurological pain can have cognitive repercussions, affecting concentration and memory. The constant battle with pain demands a significant amount of mental energy, leaving individuals fatigued and mentally strained.

5. Social Isolation:

The invisible nature of neurological pain can lead to misunderstandings and skepticism from others. This, coupled with the challenges of participating in social activities, can contribute to feelings of isolation and loneliness.

Understanding neurological pain involves recognizing its varied forms within the context of conditions like MS, Parkinson's, and fibromyalgia. Equally important is acknowledging the far-reaching consequences of pain on the overall well-being of individuals.

Chair Yoga Poses for Pain Relief

Let's explore some chair yoga poses designed to give you a sense of relief from those specific areas of discomfort. Whether it's that persistent ache or those moments of tension, these gentle stretches and movements, paired with some soothing breathing techniques, might become your go-to toolkit for pain management.

1. Neck Release:

- Place your feet firmly on the floor and settle into your chair. Lengthening your spine, inhale.
- Bring your ear to your shoulder and slightly tilt your head to one side as you release the breath.
- On the other side of your neck, feel the stretch.
- Hold for a few breaths, then switch to the other side. This one's perfect for those moments when your neck needs a little love.

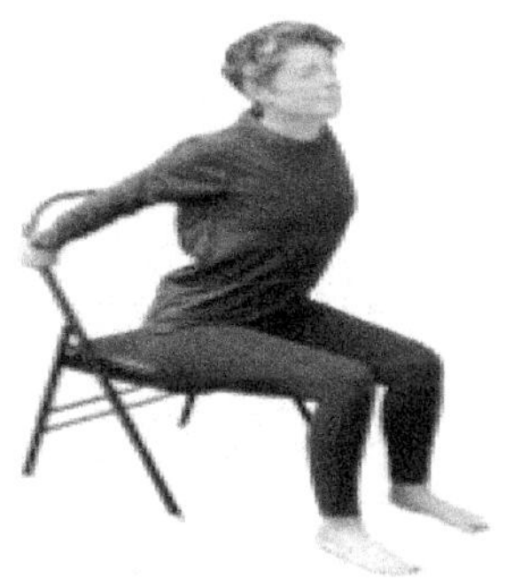

2. Seated Forward Bend:

- Move to the edge of your chair while seated.

- Lengthen your spine with an inhaled breath, then release it by hinging at the hips and extending your hands downward.
- Allow your chest to come forward, feeling a gentle stretch along your lower back and hamstrings.
- Hold for a few breaths, then slowly come back up. It's like a mini-massage for your lower back.

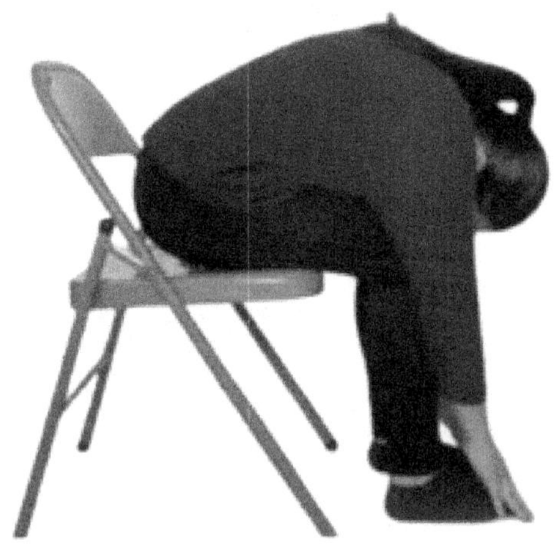

3. Seated Cat-Cow Stretch:

- Take a breath, raise your chest, and arch your back (Cow). Breathe while bringing your chin to your chest and rounding your spine (Cat).
- Exhale, rounding your spine and bringing your chin to your chest (Cat).
- Repeat this flowing movement with your breath, feeling the stretch and release in your spine. It's a subtle but effective way to alleviate tension in your back.

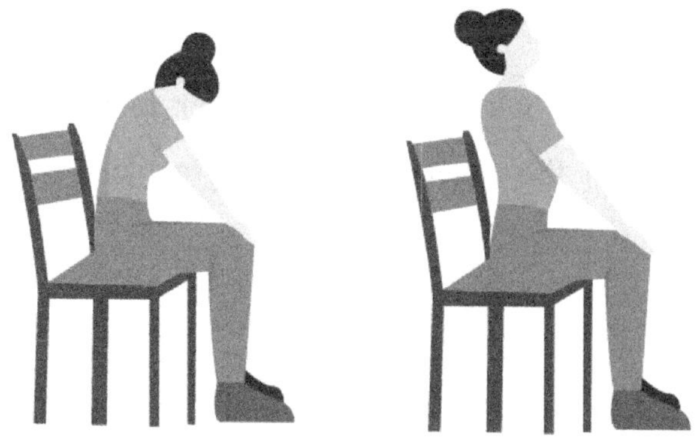

4. Wrist and Forearm Stretch:

- Extend your arms in front of you, palms facing down.
- With one hand, gently press the fingers of the other hand towards you, feeling a stretch in your wrist and forearm.
- Hold for a few breaths, then switch sides. Perfect for those moments when your wrists need a break.

5 Seated Side Stretch:

- Inhale and lift your arms overhead, clasping your hands.
- Lean gently to one side, feeling the stretch along your side of the body.
- Hold a few breaths, then come back to the center and repeat on the other side. It's a great way to release tension in your torso.

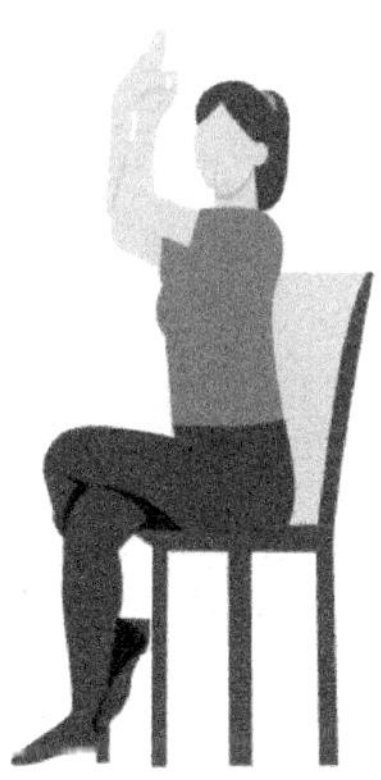

Breathing Techniques for Pain Management

1. Diaphragmaic Breathing:

- Take a comfortable seat with your hands on your stomach and chest.
- Breathe deeply through your nose and feel your tummy rise. Feel your belly drop as you gently release the breath through pursed lips.
- Concentrate on this deliberate, deep breathing to relax your nervous system and control your discomfort.

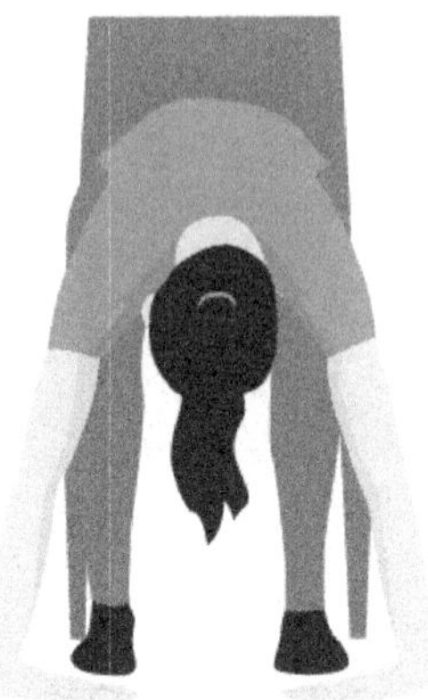

2. Box Breathing:

- Inhale for a count of four, hold your breath for four counts, exhale for four counts, and pause for another four counts before inhaling again.
- Repeat this rhyt mic pattern. It's like creating a tranquil rhythm for your breath, promoting relaxation.

3. Alternate Nostril Breathing:

- Shut one nostril with your thumb, then take a deep breath through the other.
- Close the second nostril with your pinky and exhale through the first nostril. Continue this alternate pattern.

It's a wonderful way to balance and soothe your nervous system.

Remember, these chair yoga poses and breathing techniques are your toolkit. Use them when you need relief, whether at your desk, in your living room, or anywhere you can find a chair. The beauty of chair yoga is its accessibility, making it a practical and effective way to manage pain. So, whenever you're ready for self-care, grab a chair, sit, and let these gentle movements and breaths work their magic. Your well-being deserves it!

The Role of Mindfulness in Pain Perception

Being mindful entails giving the current moment your undivided attention. Now, when it comes to pain, it's not about making the pain disappear magically. Instead, it's about changing your relationship with it. Mindfulness can alter the way you perceive and respond to pain.

Imagine this: You're sitting with a sensation of discomfort, but instead of letting your mind spiral into worry or frustration, you bring your attention to the sensation itself. By doing this, you're acknowledging the pain without letting it take over your thoughts and emotions. It's like observing a passing cloud without catching up in the storm.

Mindfulness doesn't eliminate pain, but it empowers you to be present with it and understand it; in doing so, you may find that the intensity lessens. It's a minor adjustment in viewpoint that may have a big impact.

Guided Meditation for Pain Relief

Now, let's talk about a practical tool within mindfulness—guided meditation. This is like a mental journey led by a calming voice and is particularly effective for pain relief.

Picture this:

- You find a quiet, comfortable space.
- You sit or lie down, closing your eyes. The guided meditation begins, gently directing your focus away from the pain.

- It might involve deep breathing, visualization, or a body scan, where you consciously relax each body part.

The beauty of guided meditation is that it guides your mind away from the discomfort, providing a mental sanctuary. As you follow the guidance, you might notice how you experience pain shift. It's not about ignoring it; it's about creating a mental space where the pain isn't the sole focus.

Guided meditation is like a calming friend accompanying you through the storm of discomfort. It doesn't promise to eliminate the pain, but it can create a sense of relief, both mentally and physically.

Example of a Guided Meditation

Body Scan Meditation

Body Scan Meditation is a gentle and effective practice that encourages deep relaxation and heightened body awareness. Guided by a soothing voice, this meditation takes you through various parts of your body, allowing you to release tension and foster a sense of calm.

Here's a more detailed explanation of the Body Scan Meditation:

- **Getting Comfortable:**

Locate a peaceful, cosy area where you may sit or lie down. If you feel comfortable doing so, close your eyes and take a few deep breaths to settle into the present moment.

- **Starting at the Toes:**

The guided meditation typically begins at the toes. The soothing voice directs your attention to the sensations in your toes, encouraging you to notice any tension or warmth. As you breathe, imagine letting go of any tightness in this area.

- **Moving Upwards:**

The meditation then progresses, systematically guiding your awareness through each part of your body. This may include the feet, ankles, calves, knees, and so on, gradually moving towards the head. With each segment, you're invited to observe any sensations, whether they are areas of comfort or places where tension is held.

- **Breath Awareness:**

Throughout the Body Scan, there is often a gentle reminder to maintain awareness of your breath. You might be encouraged to breathe into specific areas of tension, imagining your breath bringing a sense of ease and release.

- **Cultivating Presence:**

The essence of Body Scan Meditation lies in cultivating a heightened sense of presence and awareness. As your attention moves through different body parts, you're invited to observe without judgment, acknowledging any sensations without trying to change them.

- **Releasing Tension:**

The guiding voice encourages a softening and release of tension. As you bring attention to each part of your body, the intention is to let go of any holding, allowing muscles to relax and the body to settle.

- **Closing the Meditation:**

The Body Scan concludes by bringing attention to the body as a whole. The soothing voice may guide you to feel the entire body now relaxed and aware. It often concludes with an invitation to carry this sense of calm into your daily life.

Body Scan Meditation offers various benefits, including stress reduction, improved sleep, and increased body awareness. Individuals can release physical tension and promote overall well-being by systematically moving through the body.

Body Scan Meditation is an invitation to reconnect with your body, fostering a gentle awareness that extends beyond the meditation session. It's a practice that encourages both relaxation and a deeper understanding of the mind-body connection.

Incorporating mindfulness for pain reduction isn't just a trend; it's a profound shift in how you approach your well-being. It's about reclaiming some control over your experience of pain and recognizing that you are more than the sensations in your body.

So, the next time pain knocks on your door, consider inviting mindfulness in. It's not a quick fix, but it's a journey worth taking—one where you learn to coexist with pain, finding moments of relief and peace.

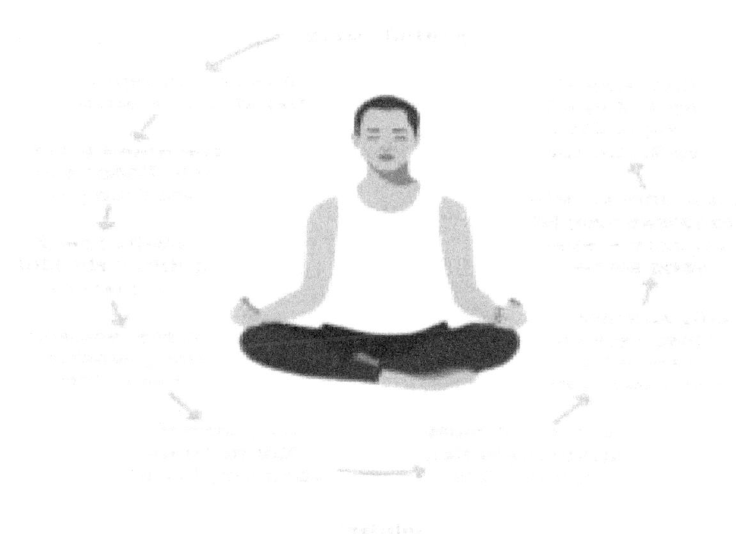

Testimony: Let me paint a picture for you—a narrative of someone who found solace in chair yoga, experiencing a remarkable reduction in pain.

Emily, a vibrant soul in her mid-40s, was no stranger to the persistent discomfort that came with fibromyalgia. The constant dull ache in her muscles had become a familiar companion, making everyday activities feel like uphill battles. The traditional exercise seemed out of reach, and finding relief felt like an elusive dream.

Enter chair yoga—a gentle, adaptable practice that met Emily where she was, both physically and emotionally. Sitting on the edge of her chair, she began with mindful breathing, grounding herself in the present moment. As the instructor guided her through gentle stretches and movements, Emily felt a sense of liberation she hadn't experienced in years.

The chair became her sanctuary, providing support and stability. Modified poses allowed her to engage muscles without the strain often accompanying traditional yoga. The rhythmic flow of chair yoga became a dance of healing for Emily, a journey inward where she could listen to her body without judgment.

As the weeks went by, Emily noticed a subtle but significant shift. The relentless grip of pain began to loosen its hold. The chair became not just a prop but a tool for empowerment. Seated twists eased tension in her spine, gentle neck stretches alleviated headaches, and slow, intentional movements became a balm for her tired muscles.

It wasn't a miraculous cure but a journey of progress—a narrative of resilience and adaptability. Emily's story became a testament to the transformative potential embedded in the mindful movements of chair yoga. She discovered a newfound sense of agency over her own well-being through consistency and compassion.

Now, Let's Take a little insight into Balance: A Pillar of Neurological Well-being which we will fully discuss about in the next chapter.

Balance exercises, often overlooked, play a pivotal role in the holistic realm of neurological well-being. It's not just about physical equilibrium; it's a dance between body and mind.

Our brain is a conductor orchestrating the symphony of movements. In neurological conditions like multiple sclerosis or Parkinson's, this symphony faces disruptions. Balance exercises step in as choreographers, helping individuals navigate the intricate dance with grace and steadiness.

Balancing on one leg, shifting weight deliberately, and practicing controlled movements aren't merely physical tasks—they're neurological workouts. They stimulate the brain's regions responsible for coordination and spatial awareness, fostering connections that neurological conditions may dull.

But the significance goes beyond the physical domain. Balance exercises create a synergy between body and mind, promoting confidence and reducing the fear of falls—a common concern for those with neurological conditions. As individuals master the art of balance, they strengthen muscles and cultivate a resilient mindset, a sense of stability that extends beyond the physical realm.

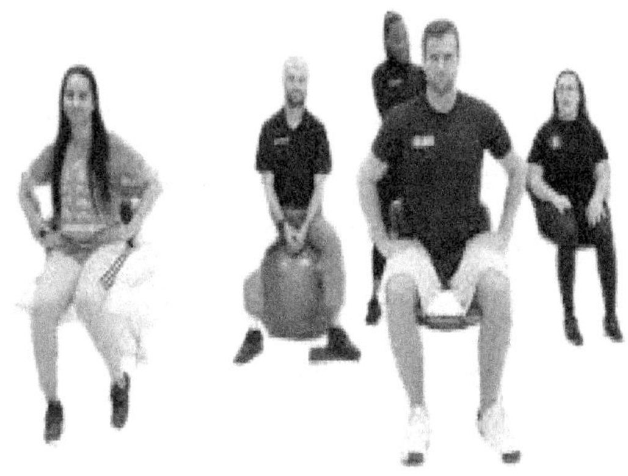

Chapter 4

Enhancing Balance for Neurological Strength

Imagine life as a delicate dance, an intricate ballet where you navigate through the ebbs and flows. In this dance, balance is not just a physical act but a metaphorical cornerstone, a guiding force that ensures harmony and stability in every step.

Just as a skilled dancer gracefully maintains equilibrium, our lives, too, require a delicate equilibrium to navigate the challenges thrown our way. This dance of life encompasses the physical realm and the intricate interplay of our thoughts, emotions, and the external world.

Picture your body as the dancer and your neurological well-being as the choreography. Just as a dancer needs a strong and stable core to execute intricate moves, your neurological system requires a foundation of balance to perform its intricate functions seamlessly.

Enhancing balance for neurological strength is akin to fine-tuning the dancer's core – it provides the stability needed for the intricate dance of signals between the brain and the body. Without balance, this dance becomes disjointed, leading to a cacophony rather than a harmonious performance.

Just as a dancer refines their technique and strengthens their core for a more graceful performance, enhancing balance for neurological strength involves intentional practices. Much like dance rehearsals, these practices can include activities that challenge and strengthen the neural pathways responsible for balance.

So, picture yourself as the lead dancer in the ballet of life, and enhancing balance for neurological strength becomes your practice session. With each intentional move, whether a mindful chair yoga pose or a gentle stretch, you fine-tun the symphony of signals within your body.

Remember, as a dancer grows stronger with each rehearsal, your neurological strength improves with consistent efforts to enhance balance. The metaphorical dance of life becomes more fluid, resilient, and in tune with the rhythm of well-being.

In this dance, balance is not just a physical act but a metaphorical cornerstone, a guiding force that ensures harmony and stability in every step. As you embark on this journey of enhancing balance for neurological strength, envision yourself dancing through life's challenges with grace and resilience, knowing that a well-balanced foundation strengthens your body and your entire being.

“Balance, the silent conductor of our body's symphony, can sometimes falter, especially in neurological conditions”.

But fear not, because here's where chair yoga steps in, becoming your trusted ally in the quest for improved balance.

Imagine the chair as your reliable anchor. In chair yoga, the support it provides becomes your stability point. Seated poses and gentle movements create a secure environment, allowing you to focus on improving balance without fearing falling.

Chair yoga introduces you to the enchanting world of mindful movement. Each deliberate stretch and pose becomes a step in strengthening your neural pathways. It's not just about physical exercise; it's a symphony of coordinated movements that enhance your body's awareness.

One size never fits all, especially in the realm of neurological conditions. Chair yoga understands this and adapts. Whether dealing with limited mobility or fatigue, chair yoga matches your needs. It's a personalized experience designed to enhance your balance at your own pace. The core, your body's centre of gravity, is like the protagonist in the balance tale. Chair yoga targets and strengthens your core muscles, the unsung heroes in the balance chronicle. As your core becomes robust, so does your ability to maintain equilibrium.

In the world of neurological conditions, confidence can sometimes waver. Chair yoga is here to uplift. As you master each pose and witness your balance improving, a newfound confidence blossoms. It's a journey of self-empowerment where every achievement becomes a testament to your strength.

One of the beauties of chair yoga is its seamless integration into your daily routine. No need for a fancy studio or elaborate props. The chair is your studio, and the movements seamlessly blend into your day. It's a practical approach that ensures consistency, a key player in the balance enhancement game.

Beyond the physical, chair yoga nurtures your mental and emotional well-being. Stress, a notorious balance disruptor, matches chair yoga's calming embrace. The holistic approach extends beyond the mat, influencing how you navigate the dance of daily life.

So, my friend, chair yoga becomes your compass, guiding you towards a more stable and confident version of yourself in the world of improving balance amidst neurological conditions. It's not just about poses; it's about reclaiming your equilibrium, one mindful movement at a time. Get ready to feel the transformative magic unfold as you embrace the chair yoga journey tailored just for you.

At the core of neurological strength lies the intricate network of neural pathways, the communication highways between the brain and the body. Balance exercises act as architects, fine-tuning these pathways with precision. When you engage in activities challenging your balance, neural signals navigate more efficiently, creating a symphony of synchronized movements.

Picture the cerebellum, a small but mighty region in your brain, as the conductor orchestrating the balanced symphony. It processes information from your senses and coordinates muscle movements. Balance exercises stimulate the cerebellum, enhancing its ability to interpret signals and execute seamless, well-coordinated actions.

Have you ever wondered how your body knows where it is in space? That's the magic of proprioception. Balance exercises sharpen this internal GPS. As you challenge your body's position, proprioceptors – specialized muscle and joint sensors – send constant feedback to the brain. This feedback loop refines your body's spatial awareness, a key component of neurological strength.

The vestibular system, nestled in your inner ear, is the unsung hero in balance. It detects head movements and changes in orientation. Balance exercises engage and optimize this system, ensuring that your body responds gracefully to shifts in position. It's like providing the balance engineer with a toolkit to maintain equilibrium.

The core muscles, encompassing the abdomen, back, and pelvis, are the pillars of support in the balanced narrative. Engaging in exercises that target core stability is akin to fortifying these pillars. A strong core provides a stable foundation, allowing the intricate dance of neural signals to unfold without unnecessary turbulence.

Balance exercises are not just about physical prowess; they're cognitive jugglers. The brain's executive functions, responsible for decision-making and multitasking, join the performance. As you navigate complex balance tasks, cognitive resilience is cultivated. This dual engagement enhances overall neurological strength, creating a dynamic interplay between body and mind.

The brain's ability to reorganize itself, known as neuroplasticity, is the true maestro behind neurological strength. Balance exercises stimulate neuroplastic changes, fostering adaptability and resilience. The brain rewires itself in response to the demands placed upon it during balance activities, sculpting a more robust and agile nervous system.

Challenges of Balance in Neurological Conditions

How conditions like Parkinson's disease impact balance.

1. The Tremors:

Picture this: You're trying to stand still, and there's this persistent, rhythmic shake in your limbs. That's the tremor, a constant companion in Parkinson's. These tremors make it challenging to keep your body steady, throwing off the delicate balance we often take for granted.

2. The Stiffness:

Now, imagine your muscles deciding to be a bit too tight, resisting the natural flow of movement. That's the stiffness that comes with Parkinson's. When your muscles are rigid, your body struggles to make those subtle adjustments needed to stay balanced.

3. The Unpredictable Freezing:

Have you ever felt your feet stuck to the ground, refusing to move forward? That's the freezing of gait. In Parkinson's, it's like hitting a sudden pause button. This unpredictable freezing can happen anytime, turning a simple step into a potential stumbling block.

4. The Challenge of Posture:

Parkinson's often comes with a change in posture. That stooped stance isn't just about appearance; it significantly affects your centre of gravity. Maintaining an upright posture becomes a conscious effort, and the shift in your body's alignment adds another layer of complexity to the balancing act.

5. The Limited Range of Motion:

Flexibility becomes a puzzle. Being flexible turns into a mystery. Your range of motion may be limited by Parkinson's disease, which can hinder your body's ability to react swiftly to positional changes.

So, what does this mean for your daily balancing act? Every step, every weight shift becomes more deliberate, a bit more calculated. It's like you're navigating a constantly changing terrain beneath your feet.

The truth is that identifying these obstacles is the first step towards figuring out how to get beyond them. It's about understanding that your body adapts to a different dance. It's not always smooth, and there might be moments of imbalance, but it's a dance you're navigating with resilience and strength.

Let's talk abou tanother important factor – the risk of falls and what it means for you. It's a topic that hits close to home, and understanding it is key to navigating your journey toward well-being.

Falls aren't just isolated incidents; they can create a chain reaction. Picture it like a line of dominoes – one fall can lead to another. The risk increases, and it becomes crucial to break this chain to maintain your overall health and quality of life.

Falls often come with the risk of injuries, not just the physical impact. There's a vulnerability that comes with it. Whether it's a bruise, a sprain, or something more severe, each injury adds a layer of complexity to your journey toward well-being.

The aftermath of a fall isn't just about the physical recovery; it's also about the emotional toll. The fear of falling again can linger, casting a shadow over daily activities. It's like a silent companion, influencing your decisions and sometimes holding you back from doing things you enjoy.

A fall that leads to hospitalization isn't just a temporary setback. It can disrupt your routine, your comfort zone, and your momentum. The recovery process might require time and effort, impacting your overall well-being.

So, what does this mean for you? It means acknowledging the reality of the situation and recognizing that falls aren't just physical events; they have broader implications. It's about understanding the potential consequences and, more importantly, taking proactive steps to minimize the risk.

Here's the thing: You're not alone in this. Strategies, exercises, and support systems are designed to enhance your stability and reduce the risk of falls. So, let's navigate this journey together – addressing the risks, embracing the solutions, and keeping your well-being at the forefront.

Chair Yoga Poses for Improved Balance

Gentle exercises promoting stability and equilibrium

Let's explore some chair yoga poses designed to enhance balance, focusing on gentle exercises promoting stability and equilibrium. Additionally, we'll discuss modifications to cater to various balance ability levels, ensuring that these poses can be adapted to your comfort and needs.

1. Seated Mountain Pose:

- Remain upright in your chair and use
- your feet flat on the floor.
- Align your spine and place your hands on your thighs.
- Take a few deep breaths, feeling grounded and stable.

Modification: Lift one foot slightly off the floor, then the other, gradually challenging your balance.

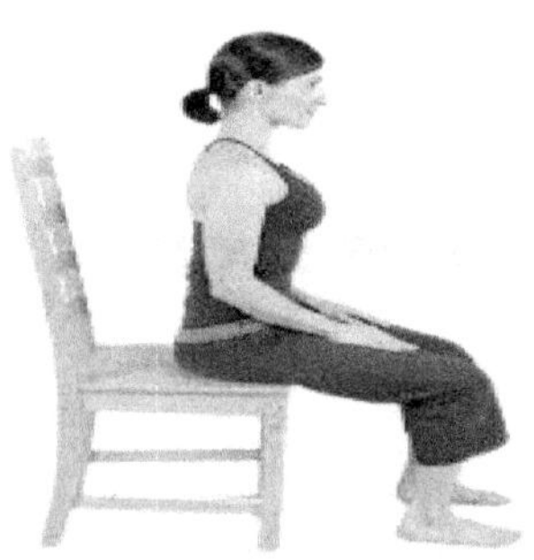

2. Seated Warrior Pose:

- Sitting, bend one leg and stretch the other straight out.
- Place the foot on the inner thigh of the extended leg.
- Reach arms overhead, stretching gently to the side.

Modification: Keep the bent knee lower or use the back of the chair for support.

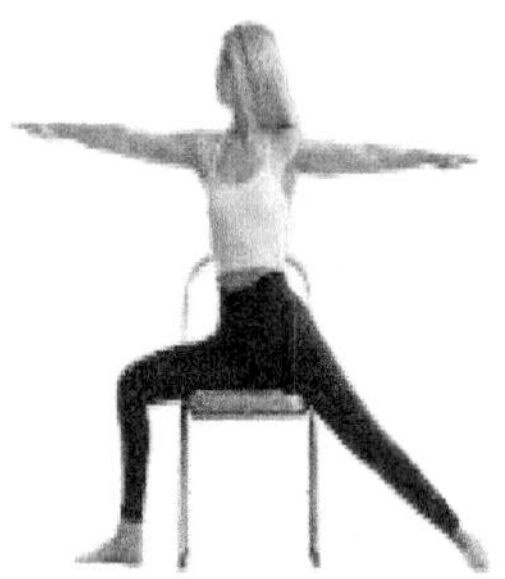

3. Seated Tree Pose:

- Sit tall, placing your right foot on the inner left thigh or calf.
- Bring palms together in front of your chest.

Modification: Keep the foot lower on the calf or use the chair for support.

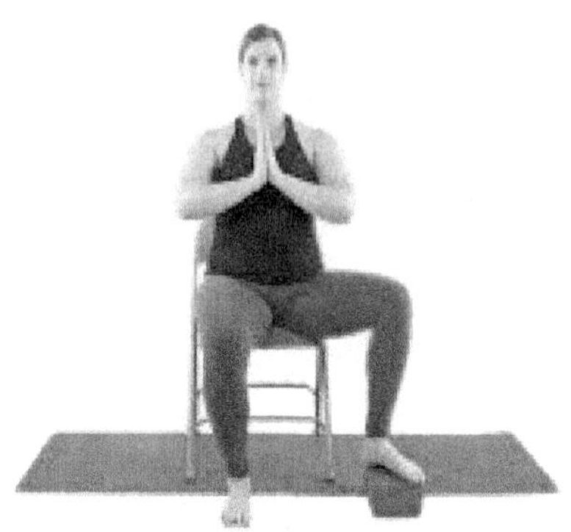

4. Seated Twist:

- Place your feet flat on the ground and sit.
- Twist your upper body to the right, placing your left hand on the right knee and right hand on the back of the chair.

Modification: Gradually deepen the twist, using the chair for support as needed.

5. Leg Extensions with Arm Reaches:

- While seated, extend one leg forward as you reach the opposite arm overhead.

- Alternate between legs and arms, focusing on controlled movements.

Modification: Start with smaller movements, gradually increasing the range of motion.

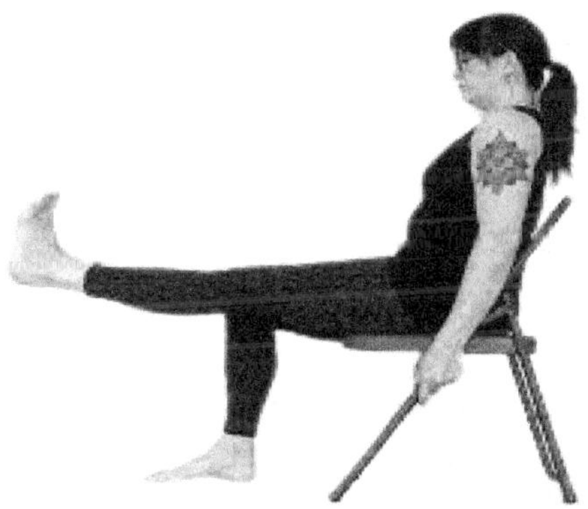

6. Seated Cat-Cow Stretch:

- Sit with a straight spine, hands on knees.
- Take a breath(Inhale), raise your chest, and arch your back (Cow Pose).
- Exhale around your spine, bringing your chin to your chest (Cat Pose).

Modification: Adjust the intensity by moderating the range of motion in both poses.

Remember: Listen to your body, progress at your own pace, and use the chair for support whenever needed. Consistent practice will gradually enhance your balance and overall well-being. Enjoy the journey!

Incorporating Strength-Building Movements

Chair yoga poses that enhance overall strength

1. Seated Chair Squats:

- Step forward of your chair with your feet hip-width apart.
- As though you were going to sit down, lower your body towards the chair and raise yourself back up.
- This mimics a squat, targeting your quadriceps, hamstrings, and glutes.

2. Seated Leg Lifts:

- Maintain a straight back when you sit at the edge of your chair.
- Lift one leg straight before you, hold it momentarily, and lower it back.
- This targets your hip flexors and strengthens your thighs.

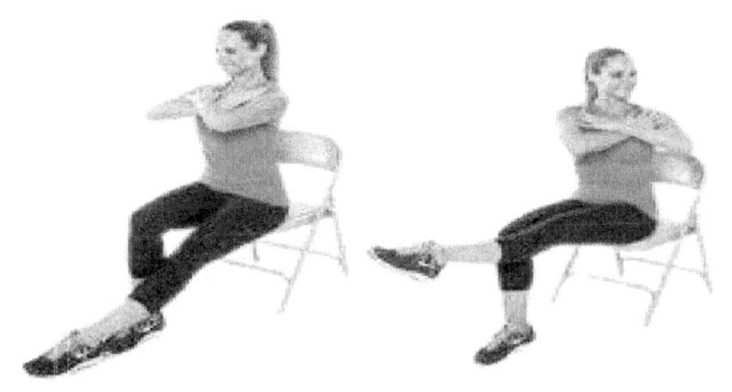

3. Seated Side Leg Raises:

- Sit tall and extend one leg out to the side.

- Lift and lower your leg, feeling the work in your outer thigh and hip.
- Switch sides and repeat. It's an excellent move for building leg strength.

4. Seated Bicep Curls:

- Hold a lightweight or a water bottle in each hand.
- Sit straight back and lift the weights towards your shoulders, engaging your biceps.
- Lower the weights back down and repeat. This strengthens your arm muscles.

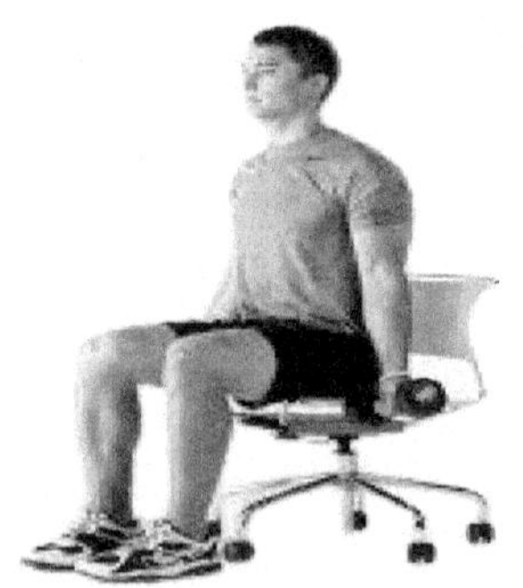

5. Seated Twist with Resistance:

- Hold a resistance band or a scarf with both hands.
- Twist your upper body to one side, then the other, feeling the resistance.
- This works on your core strength and promotes flexibility.

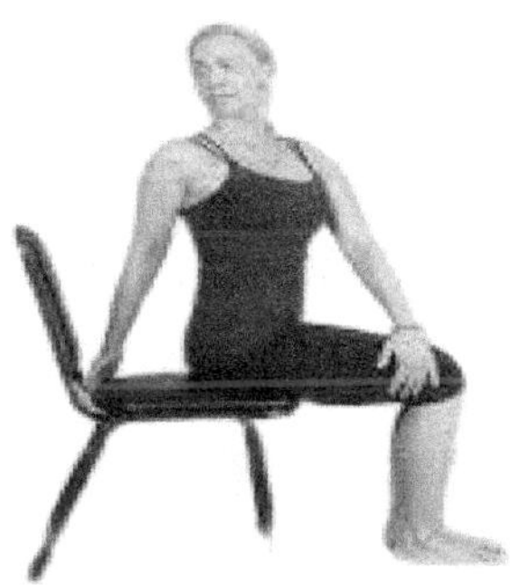

The beauty of chair yoga is its adaptability. You may adjust these motions to fit your comfort and strength level. Gradually incorporate these into your routine, focusing on controlled, deliberate movements. Building strength is a journey, and with chair yoga, it becomes a journey tailored just for you. Enjoy the process!

The relationship between strength and improved neurological well-being.

Let's dive into something powerful – the connection between building strength and boosting your neurological well-being. It's a journey that's uniquely yours, and here's why it matters:

1. Empowering Your Muscles, Empowering Your Mind:

When you engage in strength-building movements, it's like sending a powerful message to your muscles. You're saying, "Hey, we've got this!" As your muscles respond and grow stronger, it creates a ripple effect beyond the physical. Your mind tunes into this empowerment, creating a positive loop of resilience and capability.

2. The Brain-Muscle Harmony:

Your brain and muscles have this incredible dance, a harmony that influences your entire nervous system. Strength training enhances this connection. Every muscle contraction transmits messages to your brain, refining its directives.

It's like fine-tuning an orchestra. This coordination is a symphony that contributes to improved neurological function.

3. Balancing the Neurotransmitters:

Strength training triggers the release of neurotransmitters like endorphins and serotonin. These are your body's natural mood enhancers. As you build strength, you're not just toning muscles; you're creating a chemical environment that fosters feelings of well-being. It's like a built-in reward system that positively influences your neurological state.

4. The Resilience Factor:

Building strength is more than just physical; it's about cultivating resilience. Your body becomes more adaptable and better equipped to handle the ups and downs. This adaptability extends to your nervous system, fostering a resilience that plays a crucial role in managing neurological conditions.

6. Confidence and Mindset:

As you witness the physical changes – feeling stronger and more capable – it's a confidence booster. This newfound confidence seeps into your mindset. You start approaching challenges with a can-do attitude. Your neurological well-being benefits from this positive mindset, creating a mental environment that supports overall health.

6. Tackling Fatigue and Boosting Energy:

Strength-building exercises combat fatigue, a common challenge in neurological conditions. They improve your endurance, giving you more Energy for daily activities. This energy boost contributes to a more vibrant neurological well-being.

Remember, this journey is uniquely yours. Whether a gentle seated workout or a more dynamic routine, it's about finding what feels right. Listen to your body, celebrate the progress, and let strength-building become a cornerstone in your path towards improved neurological well-being.

So, here's to the strength within you, the resilience you're building, and the positive impact on your neurological well-being. It's a journey of empowerment, and you're at the helm. Keep moving forward – one strength-building moment at a time!

Chapter 5

Building Comprehensive Strength through Mindful Movement

As the ancient saying goes, "Strength is not just in the lift, but in the stillness that follows." This quote sets the tone for our exploration, hinting at the profound strength found in the quiet moments of mindful movement.

Now, let's unravel why building strength through chair yoga exercises is more than just a workout but it's a tailored approach to support your neurological well-being.

In the midst of a busy world, there's a power in stillness. It's not about lifting heavy weights or pushing your body to extremes; it's about the intentional, mindful movements that build strength from within. Just like a tree with deep roots stands firm against the wind, cultivating inner strength through mindful stillness fortifies you against life's challenges.

Chair yoga is not your typical gym session; it's a mindful ally in your journey to strengthen not just the body but the intricate connection between body and mind. In the gentle flow of chair yoga exercises, there's a dance of breath, movement, and awareness.

Chair yoga engages your muscles with intention. It's not about pushing hard; it's about activating each muscle mindfully. This focused approach brings awareness to the subtleties of movement, fostering a deeper connection between your nervous system and muscles. The intricate coordination between your brain and muscles is like a dance. Chair yoga, with its mindful sequences, fine-tunes this coordination. Each movement becomes a conversation between your mind and body, contributing to improved neuromuscular function.

The beauty of chair yoga lies in its adaptability. Whether you're a beginner or dealing with specific neurological challenges, each pose is an opportunity to build strength at your pace. It's not a race; it's a journey tailored to your unique needs.

Neurological well-being isn't just about physical strength; it's also about managing stress. Chair yoga incorporates mindfulness techniques that act as a balm for your nervous system. As you move with awareness, stress melts away, creating a positive environment for neurological health.

In essence, building comprehensive strength through mindful movement, especially in the context of chair yoga, is about embracing the power found in stillness, in intentional breaths, and in the mindful engagement of muscles. It's a journey where strength isn't just a destination; it's a continuous, mindful exploration of your body's capabilities, contributing to a resilient and empowered neurological well-being. So, let's embark on this journey together!

Imagine your body as a finely tuned instrument, and each muscle group as a crucial player in the symphony of your daily life. Comprehensive strength is like the conductor of this orchestra, ensuring that each muscle plays its part harmoniously. Comprehensive strength orchestrates the seamless coordination of your muscles, enabling a symphony of movement in your everyday activities.

From standing up to reaching for an item on a shelf, each movement requires a delicate balance between muscle groups. When neurological conditions disrupt this harmony, comprehensive strength becomes a vital ally in restoring balance and maintaining fluidity in your motions.

Simple tasks that we often take for granted, like getting out of bed, walking, or lifting groceries, can become intricate challenges when neurological conditions are in play. Comprehensive strength acts as a reliable support system, providing the muscular strength needed to execute these tasks with greater ease and reduced strain.

Neurological conditions, including Fibromyalgia, can bring about heightened fatigue. Comprehensive strength acts as a shield against this fatigue, distributing the workload among various muscle groups. Imagine it as a team effort where no single muscle is overburdened, allowing you to conserve energy for the activities that matter most.

The ability to independently perform daily tasks contributes significantly to your overall well-being. Comprehensive strength is your ally in maintaining independence by ensuring that your muscles, from the core to the limbs, are strong enough to handle the demands of daily life. This independence, in turn, fosters a sense of empowerment and autonomy.

Pain can be a constant companion for you as a Fibromyaglia patient. Comprehensive strength plays a pivotal role in mitigating pain by promoting proper alignment and reducing strain on sensitive areas. Strengthening the muscles surrounding joints provides essential support, potentially alleviating discomfort associated with conditions like Fibromyalgia.

Neurological conditions like Fibromyalgia can often compromise balance and stability. Comprehensive strength, especially in the core and lower body muscles, acts as a stabilizing force. It's the invisible thread that helps you stand tall, walk with confidence, and navigate your environment more securely.

Life with Fibromyalgia involves navigating unpredictabilities. Comprehensive strength cultivates adaptability and resilience. It's not just about lifting weights; it's about preparing your body to respond effectively to the ever-changing demands of daily life, creating a foundation for resilience in the face of challenges.

The Relationship Between Strength and Pain Management

Now, let's spotlight the unique relationship between strength and pain management in the context of Fibromyalgia. Picture strength as a shield – not just a physical one but a holistic defense mechanism against the waves of discomfort.

- **Balancing the Load:**

Comprehensive strength ensures that the workload is distributed evenly across your body. Think of it as each muscle sharing the burden, preventing certain areas from becoming overtaxed and triggering pain responses.

- **Supporting Proper Posture:**

A strong core and back muscles act like a backbone, quite literally. They support your posture, preventing unnecessary strain on your spine. This is crucial in Fibromyalgia, where maintaining a balanced posture can alleviate pain associated with misalignment.

- **Promoting Flexibility and Range of Motion:**

Strength isn't just about power; it's also about flexibility. Gentle chair yoga movements designed to enhance flexibility play a key role. When your muscles are supple, they're less prone to stiffness and the accompanying pain.

- **Mind-Body Harmony for Pain Perception:**

Comprehensive strength isn't solely physical; it's also about the mind-body connection. As you engage in strengthening movements, the relationship between your brain and muscles becomes more attuned. This mindfulness contributes to a positive environment, potentially influencing how your brain perceives and manages pain signals.

Chair Yoga Poses for Targeted Strength

Exercises targeting different muscle groups.

1. Seated Mountain Pose:

Targeted Muscles: Core, Back, Shoulders

- Sit tall in your chair, feet flat on the floor.
- As you inhale, reach your arms overhead, palms facing each other.
- Engage your core and feel the stretch along your spine.
- Exhale as you lower your arms. This gentle move strengthens your core and supports your back, areas that often bear the brunt of Fibromyalgia's effects.

2. Seated Leg Lifts:

Targeted Muscles: Quadriceps, Hamstrings

- While seated, extend one leg at a time, lifting it off the ground. Feel the engagement in your thigh muscles.

- Lower the leg and switch.

This exercise is a subtle yet effective way to strengthen your leg muscles without causing unnecessary strain.

3. Seated Twist with Resistance:

Targeted Muscles: Core, Obliques

- Sit at the edge of your chair, holding a resistance band or scarf.
- Inhale, then exhale as you twist gently from side to side. Feel the resistance in your core and oblique muscles.

This not only builds strength but also promotes flexibility in the spine.

4. Seated Bicep Curls:

Targeted Muscles: Biceps, Shoulders

- Hold light weights or water bottles in each hand.
- As you sit comfortably, curl the weights toward your shoulders, then lower them.

This simple yet effective move targets your arm muscles, promoting strength without unnecessary strain.

5. Chair Squats:

Targeted Muscles: Quadriceps, Hamstrings, Glutes

- Stand in front of your chair, feet hip-width apart.
- Lower your body as if sitting down, then stand back up.
- This mimics a squat and works wonders for your lower body muscles. Feel free to adjust the depth based on your comfort.

The Role of Breath and Mindfulness:

Now, let's not forget the breath—a constant companion in our journey. As you move through these poses, sync each movement with a mindful breath. Inhale as you prepare, exhale as you engage. This connection enhances your awareness, fostering a mindful approach to strength-building.

- **Focus on the Present:** Direct your attention to the sensations in your body as you move. Be present in each moment, acknowledging the strength you're cultivating.
- **Breathe Through Discomfort:** If you feel discomfort, breathe into it. Imagine your breath soothing the areas of tension. This mindful approach can make the exercises more manageable.

- **Celebrate Small Wins:** Every movement is a victory. Celebrate the strength you're building, no matter how subtle it may seem. This journey is about progress, not perfection.

Incorporate these chair yoga poses into your routine, honoring your body's unique needs. Let each breath and movement be a gentle reminder of the resilience within you. Remember, the key is not to rush. These movements are your tools for cultivating strength gradually. Each one is a step towards comprehensive strength, supporting you in your daily activities and contributing to effective pain management, especially in the context of neurological conditions like Fibromyalgia.

Incorporating Variety in Strength Training

Alright, imagine our strength training journey as a playlist, and chair yoga is our favorite genre. Now, this playlist can have different vibes to suit your goals—whether you're in the mood for a gentle stretch or a targeted muscle workout.

Some days, it's all about easy vibes. We'll pick poses like Seated Mountain or Leg Lifts—simple yet effective, like your favorite chill tunes. They give your muscles a nod without going full-on workout mode. Now, if you're feeling like targeting specific areas, it's like creating a custom playlist. Poses such as Seated Twist with Resistance or Seated Bicep Curls become the main tracks. It's like saying, "Hey, let's give some extra love to these muscles today."

Then, there are days when we want the whole shebang. That's where Chair Squats come into play. It's like playing your favorite upbeat song that gets your entire body moving. Engaging quads, hamstrings, and glutes—all in one go.

Remember, this is your playlist, and you get to choose the beats based on how you're feeling. If a pose feels a bit much, it's like skipping a song. No pressure, just the rhythm of your own journey.

Strength, Balance, and Weight Management

Now, let's talk about the trio—strength, balance, and weight management. It's like the core tracks that make our playlist memorable.

As we groove through our chair yoga routine, we're building a solid rhythm of balance. Strengthening the core, legs, and arms is like creating a melody that supports your balance, making you feel more grounded and sure-footed.

Strength is the bassline in our playlist. Chair yoga, with its purposeful moves, is like boosting the metabolism—your body's dance to keep things in check. It's not about heavy lifting; it's about creating a steady rhythm that contributes to a healthy relationship between movement and weight.

In this music analogy, think of mindfulness as the DJ. It's what ties everything together, making sure each beat is in sync with how you're feeling. It's not just about going through the motions; it's about feeling the rhythm, being present in each movement.

So, let's keep this playlist of chair yoga diverse, flexible, and entirely yours. It's not about perfection—it's about enjoying the tunes of your strength journey. You're the composer, the DJ, and the dancer.

Sarah's story as we have told in the introduction is one of resilience and gradual empowerment. Living with a neurological condition that affected her mobility, she found herself facing daily challenges that seemed insurmountable. Simple tasks became hurdles, and the loss of mobility took a toll on both her physical and emotional well-being.

Enter chair yoga—a beacon of hope that Sarah stumbled upon during her quest for solutions. Initially hesitant, she decided to give it a try, seeking solace in the adaptability and gentleness of the practice. Little did she know that this decision would mark a turning point in her life.

Starting with the basics, Sarah embraced the chair yoga routine with an open heart. Seated Mountain became her anchor, and Leg Lifts, her gentle victory. Each pose, carefully designed for accessibility, allowed her to engage muscles that had long been dormant.

As weeks turned into months, Sarah noticed a subtle but profound shift. The strength she thought she had lost started to awaken. Seated Twist with Resistance became a symbol of her newfound resilience, and Seated Bicep Curls transformed into a testament of her growing physical capability.

Yet, it wasn't just about the physical gains. Sarah discovered an unexpected ally in the mindfulness woven into each movement. The breath became her guide, and the present moment, her sanctuary. Chair yoga wasn't merely a series of poses; it became a holistic experience—a blend of movement, breath, and awareness.

Sarah's journey wasn't without its challenges. Some days were tougher than others, but the adaptability of chair yoga allowed her to tailor the practice to her unique needs. It was a journey of progress, not perfection.

Fast forward, and the changes in Sarah's life are palpable. The chair yoga routine, once a series of unfamiliar poses, has become her daily ritual—a source of strength, stability, and a touchstone for her overall well-being.

Now, when Sarah shares her story, it's not just about increased strength and mobility; it's a narrative of empowerment. Chair yoga became the catalyst for a positive transformation, proving that even in the face of physical challenges, one can find strength, mobility, and a renewed sense of joy. Sarah's journey is an inspiration, echoing the sentiment that sometimes, the path to strength begins with a single, mindful breath.

Once again Imagine your body as a complex orchestra with different sections—strings, woodwinds, brass, and percussion, each representing various muscle groups. Comprehensive strength acts as the conductor, guiding these sections to play in harmony. It ensures that muscles work together seamlessly, much like musicians following the lead of a conductor in a symphony.

The symphony metaphor extends to the quality of movement. Comprehensive strength allows for fluidity in motion, akin to a musical piece flowing seamlessly from one note to the next. When muscles are well-coordinated and balanced, the body moves with grace, reducing stiffness and promoting a smooth, uninterrupted flow in daily activities.

In a symphony, each instrument plays a unique role, contributing to the overall composition. Similarly, each muscle group has its function in movement. Comprehensive strength ensures that these muscles work in tandem, efficiently supporting one another. This collaborative effort enhances the efficiency of movements, making activities like walking, reaching, or lifting more effortless.

Just as a well-conducted symphony minimizes discordant sounds, comprehensive strength minimizes strain and tension in the body. When muscles are balanced and strengthened, they share the workload, preventing any single muscle group from becoming overburdened. This orchestration reduces the risk of strain or discomfort during daily tasks.

A symphony adapts to the conductor's cues, responding to changes in tempo or dynamics. Similarly, comprehensive strength equips the body with the ability to adapt to various challenges. Whether it's navigating uneven terrain or reaching for an object, a well-coordinated symphony of muscles ensures an adaptive and responsive movement.

Like musicians attuned to the conductor's guidance, comprehensive strength enhances body awareness. Individuals with well-developed strength have a heightened sense of how their body moves in space. This awareness is crucial for maintaining balance, preventing falls, and ensuring a confident and controlled execution of daily activities.

This strength is like a reliable support system, helping you with everyday tasks, from getting out of bed to lifting groceries. It's the muscular foundation that makes these tasks easier, reducing strain and making daily life more manageable. We know fatigue can be a major player in the Fibromyalgia game. Comprehensive strength is like your ally against this. It smartly spreads the workload among your muscles, preventing any single muscle from getting too tired. This balanced approach helps you conserve energy for what truly matters, ensuring a more sustainable routine and lessening the impact of fatigue.

Independence is gold, right? Comprehensive strength is your key to maintaining it. By making sure your muscles, from your core to your limbs, are strong and ready for action, it empowers you to handle the demands of daily life. It's like having the strength to say, "I've got this," fostering a sense of empowerment and autonomy.

Pain is a tough companion, but comprehensive strength can help ease its grip. It promotes proper alignment, reduces strain on sensitive areas, and strengthens muscles that support your joints. Think of it as a shield against pain, making movement more comfortable and giving you a better shot at pain relief.

Balance can be a bit tricky with Fibromyalgia, right? Comprehensive strength, especially in your core and lower body muscles, acts like a stabilizing force. It helps you stand tall, walk with confidence, and move around more securely. It's like having a built-in support system to navigate your environment with increased stability.

Life with Fibromyalgia comes with its share of uncertainties. Comprehensive strength is your secret weapon, fostering adaptability and resilience. It's not just about lifting weights; it's about preparing your body to handle the unpredictable challenges life throws your way. It's your way of saying, "I'm ready for whatever comes."

In a nutshell, building comprehensive strength is your journey towards holistic well-being. It's not just about muscles; it's about embracing the interconnected nature of your body and mind. Think of it as your silent ally, working behind the scenes to foster strength, balance, and vitality in the face of Fibromyalgia. You've got this!

CHAPTER 6:

Gentle Stretches for Daily Flexibility

Imagine your body as a book, and each gentle stretch is a page turning, allowing your story to unfold with more ease and comfort. In the world of Fibromyalgia, where each day can feel like a new chapter, these gentle stretches become your tools for adapting to life's twists and turns.

Flexibility is like the secret sauce that helps you navigate the pages of your story smoothly. It's the ability to bend and sway, just like a tree in a gentle breeze, without breaking. In the grand tale of living with Fibromyalgia, flexibility becomes your trusted companion, letting you move through the narrative of each day with grace and adaptability.

Now, picture each gentle stretch as a pause in your story, a moment to breathe and unfold the next chapter with a little more flexibility. It's not about pushing too hard or rushing through; it's about giving your body the gentle care it deserves.

Your daily flexibility routine becomes a sequence of these gentle stretches, each one a note in the melody of your day. From the soft opening stretch that greets the morning sun to the calming stretches that usher in the evening, these movements become your daily companions, adding a soothing rhythm to your journey with Fibromyalgia.

Life loves to surprise us with unexpected plot twists, and living with Fibromyalgia is no exception. Gentle stretches act as your plot armor, helping you adapt to these twists with a little more ease. Just as a well-stretched rubber band is less likely to snap, your gently stretched muscles become more resilient to the unexpected challenges that may arise.

Once again think of your body as a cherished book, and each gentle stretch as a page of self-care. It's not just about physical flexibility; it's about nurturing your body, turning each page with intention, and allowing your story with Fibromyalgia to unfold with a sense of comfort and self-compassion.

The Significance of Gentle Stretches in Improving Daily Flexibility

Living with Fibromyalgia often means navigating a unique landscape of sensitivities and challenges. Gentle stretches, like soft whispers to your muscles, hold a special significance in enhancing your daily flexibility.

1. Easing the Tension: Fibromyalgia can bring a symphony of tension to your body, like a melody that plays in the background. Gentle stretches act as the soothing notes, gradually easing the tension that can build up in muscles. It's not about pushing boundaries but coaxing your body into a state of comfort.

2. Unwinding the Knots: Imagine your muscles as intricately tied knots. Gentle stretches are like patient fingers delicately working to untangle these knots. They offer a gradual and tender release, promoting a sense of relief and making movements less cumbersome.

3. Enhancing Blood Flow: Gentle stretches encourage a gentle flow of blood through your muscles. This increased circulation is like a gentle stream carrying essential nutrients to different parts of your body. It brings a subtle warmth, offering a comforting sensation and aiding in the relaxation of tense muscles.

4. Promoting Joint Flexibility: Your joints may sometimes feel like well-worn hinges that need a bit of care. Gentle stretches provide that care, enhancing the flexibility of your joints. It's like giving your body the room it needs to move more freely, making daily activities less rigid and more comfortable.

5. Creating a Mind-Body Connection: Fibromyalgia isn't just about the physical; it weaves into the fabric of your emotions and mental well-being. Gentle stretches become a bridge, connecting your mind and body. As you engage in these mindful movements, it's a moment of self-awareness, a pause to acknowledge and care for both your physical and emotional self.

6. Improving Sleep Quality: The calming nature of gentle stretches can extend beyond the stretching session. Many find that incorporating these stretches into a bedtime routine contributes to better sleep quality. It's a gentle lullaby for your body, inviting it to relax and unwind, paving the way for a more restful night.

7. Empowering Self-Care: In the tapestry of self-care, gentle stretches become a fundamental thread. They are your personal toolkit for nurturing your body, providing a tangible way to engage in self-care. Each stretch is a moment of self-compassion, a small act of kindness toward your body.

8. Tailored to Your Pace: Gentle stretches honor your body's unique rhythm. There's no rush, no force. They are designed to be adaptable to your pace, ensuring that you have the freedom to move in a way that feels right for you on any given day.

In essence, these gentle stretches hold the power to be a daily ritual of self-love, a way to care for your body with the tenderness it deserves in the narrative of living with Fibromyalgia.

The Impact of Neurological Conditions on Flexibility

Living with Fibromyalgia, it's like your muscles are the storytellers of your experiences, and flexibility is a crucial aspect of their narrative.

Neurological conditions like Fibromyalgia can heighten the sensitivity of your muscles. It's as if your muscle fibers become delicate strings in a symphony, reacting more intensely to the notes of movement. This heightened sensitivity can sometimes lead to stiffness and a feeling of resistance.

Picture pain perception as a puzzle, and neurological conditions introduce some unexpected pieces. The signals between your nerves and brain, which usually coordinate smoothly, might encounter disruptions. This puzzle-like challenge can contribute to a sense of tightness and reduced flexibility as your muscles navigate this altered communication.

Tension becomes a dance partner in this narrative. Neurological conditions may influence the way your muscles hold onto tension, almost like a dance that's difficult to break free from. This persistent tension can create knots and reduce the natural elasticity of your muscles, impacting their ability to stretch and move with ease.

Fatigue, another character in the story, often takes center stage in neurological conditions like fibromyaglia. Muscles that are fatigued tend to resist movement, akin to tired actors on a stage. This resistance can make it challenging for your muscles to fully embrace the stretches and movements that contribute to flexibility.

In the intricate dialogue between your nervous system and muscles, neurological conditions can introduce moments of miscommunication. It's like the lines of a phone call getting crossed, leading to confusion. This miscommunication can manifest as challenges in coordinating smooth, flexible movements.

Understanding how neurological conditions affect flexibility is like embarking on a quest for gentle guidance. It involves recognizing the unique ways in which your muscles respond to movement and acknowledging that the path to flexibility may need to be paved with patience and understanding.

As a Fibromyalgia patient, it's about embracing a concept of adaptive flexibility. This means recognizing that flexibility might not always look the same for everyone, and that's perfectly okay. It's about finding movements and stretches that honor your body's unique rhythm, allowing for flexibility in a way that feels right for you.

In essence, the impact of neurological conditions on flexibility is a multifaceted tale, and understanding it involves acknowledging the intricacies of how your muscles respond to the narrative of movement. It's about navigating this story with compassion, adapting your approach, and recognizing that flexibility, in its many forms, is still a part of your journey.

How Fibromyalgia Affects Muscle Flexibility

Living with Fibromyalgia introduces a unique dynamic to the way your muscles move and stretch. Here's a closer look at how this condition may influence your muscle flexibility:

1. Heightened Sensitivity: Fibromyalgia often heightens the sensitivity of your muscles. Imagine your muscles as finely tuned instruments; with Fibromyalgia, they become more responsive to stimuli. This heightened sensitivity can sometimes result in a feeling of tightness and reluctance to fully engage in certain movements.

2. Increased Tension and Knots: Persistent tension is a common companion in Fibromyalgia. It's like your muscles are engaged in an ongoing tug-of-war, holding onto tension that can manifest as knots. These knots can limit the natural flexibility of your muscles, making it challenging to achieve the full range of motion.

3. Pain Perception Challenges: Pain perception becomes a puzzle affected by Fibromyalgia. The signals between your nerves and brain, responsible for interpreting pain, may encounter disruptions. This altered pain perception can contribute to a sense of discomfort and a hesitancy to engage in activities that involve stretching and movement.

4. Fatigue's Influence on Flexibility: Fatigue often takes center stage in Fibromyalgia. Muscles that are fatigued may resist movement, leading to a sense of stiffness. This resistance can impact your ability to engage in activities that promote flexibility, as your muscles may be less willing to respond to the demands of stretching.

5. Challenges in Communication: The communication between your nervous system and muscles may experience occasional hiccups. It's like a conversation where the lines get crossed, resulting in moments of miscommunication. This can affect the coordination of movements, making it more challenging to achieve smooth and flexible actions.

6. Adaptation and Patience: Understanding how Fibromyalgia affects muscle flexibility involves a process of adaptation and patience. It means recognizing that your body may respond differently to movement, and that's okay. It's about finding a balance between gentle encouragement and allowing your muscles the time they need to adapt to stretches and movements.

7. Individualized Approach to Flexibility: Flexibility in the context of Fibromyalgia becomes a highly individualized concept. It involves discovering what movements work best for your body, acknowledging any limitations, and embracing a flexible approach that honors your unique experience with this condition.

In essence, as a Fibromyalgia patient, the impact on muscle flexibility is a nuanced interplay of sensitivity, tension, pain perception, and the need for adaptability. It's a journey that invites you to explore what flexibility means for you and to approach it with the understanding that your body may respond in its own unique way.

The Role of Stretching in Alleviating Stiffness

Living with Fibromyalgia often involves navigating the challenges of stiffness, a sensation that can impact your day-to-day comfort. Stretching becomes a valuable tool in your self-care toolkit, offering a way to alleviate and manage this stiffness effectively.

Here's how stretching plays a crucial role:

1. Increasing Blood Flow: Stretching gently increases blood flow to the muscles. Improved circulation brings a fresh supply of oxygen and nutrients to the muscle tissues, promoting relaxation. This increased blood flow acts as a natural countermeasure to the stiffness often experienced in Fibromyalgia.

2. Loosening Tight Muscles: Stretching encourages the muscles to lengthen and relax. Tight muscles, often a source of stiffness, can benefit from the gentle elongation that stretching provides. It's like giving your muscles permission to release tension, allowing them to soften and become more pliable.

3. Enhancing Flexibility and Range of Motion: Regular stretching gradually improves flexibility and range of motion. For someone with Fibromyalgia, where stiffness can limit movement, this increased flexibility becomes particularly valuable. It allows you to move more freely, perform daily activities with greater ease, and reduces the feeling of being "locked up."

4. Promoting Mind-Body Connection: Stretching is not just a physical practice; it's also an opportunity to connect with your body on a deeper level. Engaging in mindful stretching brings attention to the sensations in your muscles. This mind-body connection can enhance your awareness of areas of tension and stiffness, allowing you to tailor your stretches to address specific needs.

5. Relieving Muscle Tension: Stiffness often accompanies heightened muscle tension. Gentle stretching serves as a mechanism to relieve this tension. As you stretch, the muscle fibers relax, and the tension gradually dissipates. It's a therapeutic process that provides relief and contributes to an overall sense of comfort.

6. Improved Joint Mobility: Stretching also benefits joint health. Fibromyalgia can sometimes affect the joints, leading to stiffness. Regular stretching helps maintain and improve joint mobility, ensuring that your joints can move through their full range without discomfort.

7. Incorporating Gentle Movements: For Fibromyalgia patients, the key is to incorporate gentle stretching movements. It's not about pushing your body to extremes but introducing stretches that respect your current level of comfort. Gentle movements allow you to gradually increase your flexibility without triggering additional discomfort.

8. Forming a Consistent Routine: Consistency is key. Regular, gentle stretching forms a foundation for managing stiffness in Fibromyalgia. Establishing a routine ensures that your muscles are regularly engaged in movements that promote flexibility, contributing to an ongoing sense of ease in your body.

In essence, stretching becomes a mindful and purposeful practice, tailored to the unique needs of someone navigating Fibromyalgia. It's a gentle, proactive approach to managing stiffness, fostering a sense of comfort, and promoting a more flexible and adaptable body.

Chair Yoga Stretches for Improved Flexibility

Ensure that you perform these stretches at a slow and controlled pace, only moving within your comfort zone. If you experience any pain or discomfort, adjust the intensity or skip that particular stretch.

1. Seated Neck Stretch:

- Sit comfortably in the chair with your spine straight.
- Inhale, then exhale and tilt your head gently to one side, bringing your ear toward your shoulder.
- Hold for 15-30 seconds, feeling a gentle stretch along the side of your neck.
- Repeat on the other side.

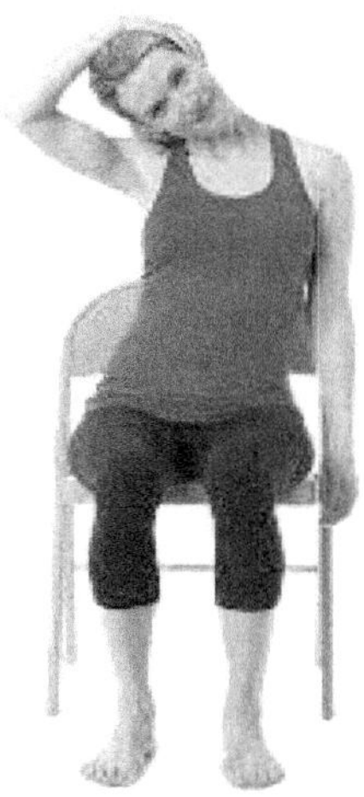

2. Shoulder Rolls:

- Sit with your back straight and shoulders relaxed.
- Inhale as you lift your shoulders up toward your ears.
- Exhale as you roll them back and down in a circular motion.
- Repeat this rolling motion for 1 minute, then reverse the direction.

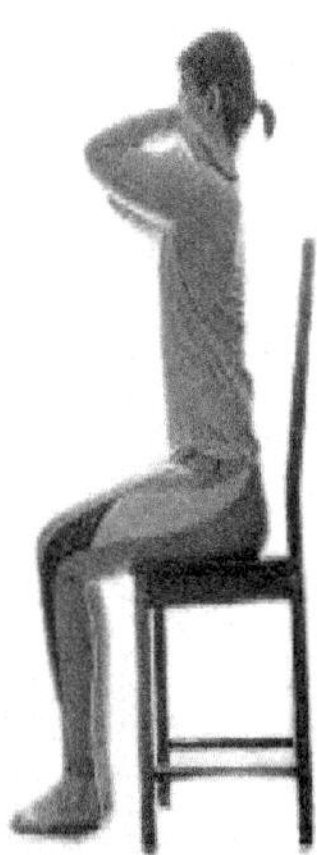

3. Seated Forward Fold:

- Sit on the edge of the chair with feet flat on the floor.
- Inhale, lengthen your spine, and as you exhale, hinge at your hips and reach forward.

- Allow your hands to reach toward the floor or rest on your shins.
- Hold for 15-30 seconds, feeling a gentle stretch along your spine and hamstrings.

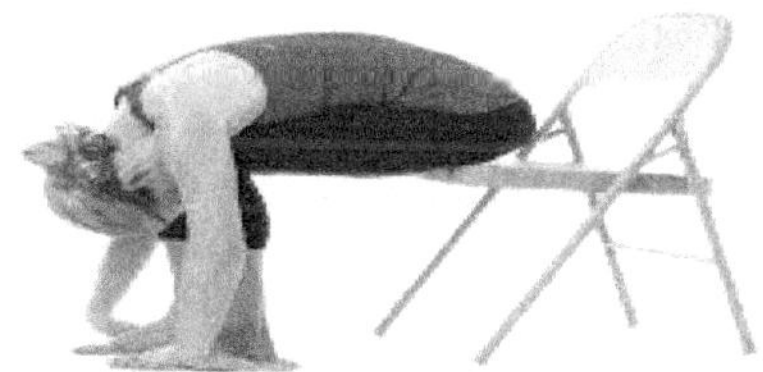

4. Seated Twist:

- Sit with your back straight and your feet flat on the floor.
- Inhale, lengthen your spine, and as you exhale, twist to one side.
- Place one hand on the outside of the opposite knee and the other hand on the back of the chair.

- Hold for 15-30 seconds, feeling a gentle twist through your spine.
- Repeat on the other side.

5. Wrist and Ankle Circles:

- Extend your arms straight in front of you and rotate your wrists clockwise and then counterclockwise for 30 seconds each.
- Lift one foot and make circles with your ankle, then switch to the other foot. Repeat for 30 seconds each.

6. Seated Cat-Cow Stretch:

- Sit with your hands on your knees.
- Inhale as you arch your back, lifting your chest and chin (Cow position).
- Exhale as you round your spine, tucking your chin to your chest (Cat position).
- Repeat this flowing movement for 1-2 minutes.

7. Seated Butterfly Stretch:

- Sit with your back straight and bring the soles of your feet together.
- Hold your feet with your hands and let your knees gently drop toward the sides.
- Hold for 15-30 seconds, feeling a gentle stretch in your inner thighs.

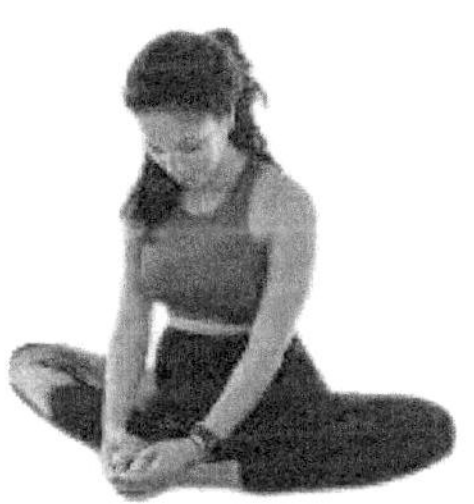

8. Seated Leg Extension:

- Sit with your back straight and extend one leg forward.
- Flex your foot and reach toward your toes, feeling a stretch in your hamstring.
- Hold for 15-30 seconds and switch to the other leg.

Remember, the key is to move gently, respecting your body's current state. If any stretch feels uncomfortable, modify or skip it. Regular practice of these chair yoga stretches can contribute to improved flexibility and overall comfort, tailored to the unique needs of someone with Fibromyalgia.

Incorporating dynamic and static stretches for optimal results.

incorporating a combination of dynamic and static stretches can be beneficial for someone with Fibromyalgia, offering a well-rounded approach to flexibility and comfort. Let's understand how you can integrate both types of stretches for optimal results:

Dynamic Stretches:

Warm-Up with Gentle Movements:

- Start your routine with 5-10 minutes of gentle movements like marching in place or light shoulder rolls.

- Dynamic movements increase blood flow, warming up your muscles and preparing them for deeper stretches.

Joint Circles:

- Perform gentle joint circles, especially for wrists, ankles, and shoulders.
- Circulating your joints through a full range of motion helps reduce stiffness and enhances joint mobility.

Dynamic Arm Swings:

- Stand or sit comfortably and swing your arms forward and backward in controlled motions.
- This helps engage your shoulder muscles and encourages flexibility in the upper body.

Leg Swings:

- Hold onto a stable surface for support and swing one leg forward and backward.
- This dynamic leg movement warms up your hips and legs, promoting flexibility.

Torso Twists:

- Sit or stand with your feet hip-width apart and twist your torso from side to side.
- Torso twists are gentle and help in warming up the spine and improving flexibility.

Transition to Static Stretches:

Neck Stretch:

- Gently tilt your head to one side, holding for 15-30 seconds.
- This static stretch allows the muscles in your neck to relax and lengthen.

Shoulder Stretch:

- Bring one arm across your chest and gently hold it with the opposite hand.
- Hold for 15-30 seconds, feeling a stretch across the shoulders.

Hamstring Stretch:

- Sit with one leg extended and gently reach toward your toes.
- Hold for 15-30 seconds, feeling a stretch in the back of your thigh.

Chest Opener:

- Clasp your hands behind your back and open your chest, squeezing your shoulder blades together.
- Hold for 15-30 seconds, stretching the chest and shoulders.

Seated Forward Fold:

- Sit on the edge of a chair and fold forward, reaching toward your toes.
- Hold for 15-30 seconds, feeling a stretch along your spine and hamstrings.

Calf Stretch:

- Stand facing a wall, place one foot behind you, and press the heel into the floor.
- Hold for 15-30 seconds, stretching the calf muscles.

Tips for Optimal Results

- Pay attention to how your body responds to each movement.
- If a stretch feels uncomfortable or causes pain, adjust or skip it.
- Start with shorter durations and gradually increase the hold time as your flexibility improves.
- Progress at a pace that feels comfortable for you.
- Incorporate stretching into your routine regularly.
- Consistent practice helps maintain and improve flexibility over time.

- Focus on deep, mindful breathing during both dynamic and static stretches.
- Controlled breathing enhances relaxation and helps release tension.

By combining dynamic movements to warm up your muscles with static stretches for deeper flexibility, you create a balanced and effective stretching routine. This approach is tailored to accommodate your unique needs promoting comfort and improved overall flexibility.

Daily Stretching Routine for Long-Term Flexibility

let's design a sustainable and manageable daily stretching routine tailored to your needs as somcone with Fibromyalgia. This routine focuses on gentle stretches and aims to promote long-term flexibility while considering the unique challenges associated with Fibromyalgia.

Note: Perform each stretch slowly and within your comfort zone. If you experience any pain, modify or skip the stretch. Consult with your healthcare provider before starting any new exercise routine.

1. Neck Stretch (Dynamic):

- Slowly tilt your head from side to side, moving in a gentle, controlled motion.
- Repeat for 1-2 minutes.

2. Shoulder Rolls (Dynamic):

- Lift your shoulders up toward your ears and roll them back in a circular motion.
- Repeat for 1-2 minutes, then reverse the direction.

3. Arm Swings (Dynamic):

- Stand or sit comfortably and swing your arms forward and backward.
- Engage in this dynamic movement for 2-3 minutes.

4. Wrist Circles (Dynamic):

- Rotate your wrists in clockwise and counterclockwise circles.
- Perform for 1 minute in each direction.

5. Seated Cat-Cow Stretch (Dynamic):

- Sit with your hands on your knees and alternate between arching and rounding your back.
- Repeat for 2-3 minutes.

6. Chest Opener (Static):

- Clasp your hands behind your back and open your chest.
- Hold for 15-30 seconds, focusing on deep breaths.

7. Seated Forward Fold (Static):

- Sit on the edge of a chair, inhale, lengthen your spine, and exhale as you fold forward.
- Hold for 15-30 seconds, feeling a gentle stretch in your hamstrings and lower back.

8. Leg Extension (Static):

- Sit with one leg extended, flex your foot, and reach toward your toes.
- Hold for 15-30 seconds and switch to the other leg.

9. Ankle Rolls (Dynamic):

- Lift one foot and make circles with your ankle.
- Rotate in both clockwise and counterclockwise directions for 1 minute, then switch to the other foot.

10. Seated Butterfly Stretch (Static):

- Sit with the soles of your feet together and hold your feet with your hands.
- Gently press your knees toward the floor, holding for 15-30 seconds.

11. Gentle Side Stretch (Static):

- r side.

12. Deep Breathing (Mindful):

- Finish your routine with 2-3 minutes of deep, mindful breathing.
- Inhale deeply through your nose, exhale through your mouth, focusing on relaxation.

Tips:

- Start with shorter durations and gradually increase as your flexibility improves.
- Perform stretches in a comfortable and quiet space.
- Listen to your body and adjust as needed.

This daily stretching routine is designed to be gentle, adaptable, and achievable for long-term flexibility. Consistency is key, so aim to incorporate these stretches into your daily routine. Always prioritize your comfort and consult with your healthcare provider if you have any concerns.

The cumulative benefits of consistent gentle stretches

Consistent gentle stretches can offer several cumulative benefits for individuals with fibromyalgia.

While every person may experience different results, here are some potential cumulative benefits you may gain from incorporating regular and gentle stretching into your routine:

- **Improved Flexibility:**

Regular stretching helps increase the range of motion in your joints and muscles. Over time, this improved flexibility can enhance your overall mobility, making daily movements more comfortable.

- **Reduced Muscle Tension:**

Gentle stretching helps release muscle tension, a common issue in fibromyalgia. Cumulatively, this may contribute to a decrease in stiffness and discomfort in the muscles.

- **Enhanced Circulation:**

Stretching promotes better blood circulation, aiding in the delivery of oxygen and nutrients to your muscles. Improved circulation may contribute to reduced fatigue and increased energy levels.

- **Stress Relief:**

Gentle stretches, especially when combined with deep breathing, can promote relaxation. Over time, this may lead to a cumulative reduction in stress levels, positively impacting overall well-being.

- **Better Posture:**

Regular stretching can help improve and maintain good posture. As your muscles become more flexible, you may find it easier to maintain proper alignment in daily activities.

- **Enhanced Joint Health:**

Gentle stretches contribute to the health of your joints by promoting lubrication and flexibility. This may lead to reduced joint discomfort over time.

- **Improved Sleep Quality:**

The relaxation benefits of consistent stretching may positively impact sleep quality. Better sleep can, in turn, contribute to improved overall health and well-being.

- **Mind-Body Connection:**

Engaging in regular stretching fosters a connection between your body and mind. Over time, this heightened awareness may help you better manage stress and pain.

- **Pain Management:**

While individual responses vary, some people with fibromyalgia report reduced pain levels with consistent stretching. The cumulative effect may lead to better pain management and an improved sense of comfort.

- **Increased Confidence:**

As you experience improvements in flexibility and reduced discomfort, you may gain confidence in your ability to manage your fibromyalgia symptoms.

It's essential to approach stretching with patience and adaptability, modifying exercises as needed based on your comfort level.

CHAPTER 7

Mindful Eating Practices for Nutritional Well-being

Did you know that the way you eat can profoundly impact your overall well-being?

Let's uncover the surprising connection between mindful eating and nutritional health, especially tailored for individuals navigating the challenges of fibromyalgia. In the journey toward better health, the role of nutrition cannot be overstated. For those with fibromyalgia, where managing symptoms is a daily consideration, adopting mindful eating practices can be a game-changer.

Fibromyalgia often intertwines with heightened sensitivity, affecting not just the body but also how we experience and respond to various stimuli, including food.

Mindful eating involves cultivating a heightened awareness of the eating experience, fostering a deeper connection with the food we consume.

Being totally present and involved during the eating process is the foundation of mindful eating. It entails enjoying the flavours, textures, and fragrances of every meal while focusing on the whole sensory experience. Eating with intention as opposed to instinctively is encouraged by mindful eating.

Spend a time setting a good intention to fuel your body with the right foods and nourishment before each meal. Both the symptoms of fibromyalgia and the way your body reacts to food might change. Pay attention to your body's distinct indications about hunger and fullness. Chew each bite carefully to slow down the eating process. This helps with digestion and lets you enjoy the tastes and textures of your meal more.

Set a comfortable and inviting space for meals, free from distractions. Creating a positive environment can enhance the overall eating experience. Fibromyalgia may impact metabolism, making portion control important. Pay attention to portion sizes and savor the quality of the food rather than focusing solely on quantity.

Use all your senses while eating—notice the colors, smells, and even the sounds of your meal. Engaging your senses promotes a holistic experience and connection with your food. Staying hydrated is crucial for overall health.

Consciously sipping water and being mindful of your body's hydration needs is an integral part of nutritional well-being. After meals, take a moment to reflect on how different foods make you feel. - This reflection can guide you in making choices that align with your well-being.

Consistent practice of mindful eating can lead to improved digestion, better nutrient absorption, and a more positive relationship with food. - For individuals with fibromyalgia, this approach fosters a harmonious connection between the body and the nourishment it receives.

Embracing mindful eating isn't just about what's on your plate; it's about fostering a relationship with your food that supports your unique journey with fibromyalgia.

Nutritional Challenges in Neurological Conditions

Navigating nutritional challenges in the context of fibromyalgia is a unique journey, and understanding these challenges is a crucial step toward developing a personalized and supportive approach.

Let's delve into some common nutritional issues associated with fibromyalgia, considering your specific needs:

1. Sensitivities and Trigger Foods:

Fibromyalgia is often linked to heightened sensitivities, and this extends to certain foods. Identifying trigger foods that may exacerbate symptoms is essential. This could include paying attention to reactions to gluten, dairy, or specific additives.

2. Digestive Discomfort:

Individuals with fibromyalgia may experience digestive issues, such as irritable bowel syndrome (IBS) or general discomfort.

Incorporating easily digestible foods and mindful eating practices can help manage digestive challenges.

3. Energy Levels and Nutrient Intake:

Fatigue is a common symptom of fibromyalgia, impacting energy levels. Maintaining a well-balanced diet rich in nutrients is crucial to provide sustained energy. This may involve focusing on nutrient-dense foods.

4. Medication Interactions:

Some medications used in the management of fibromyalgia symptoms may interact with certain nutrients. It's important to be aware of potential interactions and, if necessary, consult with healthcare providers to adjust nutritional intake accordingly.

5. Weight Management:

Fibromyalgia can influence weight, with individuals experiencing weight gain or loss.

Establishing a balanced and individualized approach to weight management is vital, considering the impact on overall well-being.

6. Hydration Challenges:

Fibromyalgia symptoms may affect hydration levels, leading to challenges in maintaining adequate fluid intake.

Implementing mindful hydration practices, such as sipping water throughout the day, is important for overall health.

7. Limited Physical Activity:

Pain and fatigue associated with fibromyalgia may limit physical activity, potentially affecting metabolism. Adjusting nutritional choices to accommodate activity levels is essential for maintaining a healthy weight.

8. Emotional Eating and Stress:

Emotional factors, including stress, can influence eating habits. Developing strategies to manage stress and mindful eating practices can contribute to a healthier relationship with food.

Fibromyalgia manifests differently in each person, necessitating an individualized approach to nutrition. Working with healthcare providers and possibly a registered dietitian can help tailor dietary recommendations to your specific needs and preferences.

Consider adopting a holistic approach to nutrition, focusing on a variety of nutrient-rich foods to support overall well-being. - Integrating anti-inflammatory foods and those promoting gut health may be beneficial.

Understanding and addressing these nutritional challenges of fibromyalgia is a dynamic process. Regular communication with healthcare providers and a personalized approach to nutrition can empower you to make choices that support your well-being on this unique journey.

The impact of nutrition on energy levels and overall health.

As a fibromyalgia patient, the impact of nutrition on your energy levels and overall health is significant. The right dietary choices can play a crucial role in managing symptoms, promoting well-being, and enhancing your quality of life.

Here's a breakdown of how nutrition can affect your energy levels and overall health:

1. Energy Levels:

- Nutrient-Dense Foods: Choosing nutrient-dense foods provides your body with essential vitamins, minerals, and energy.
- Balanced Meals: Consuming well-balanced meals, including a mix of carbohydrates, proteins, and healthy fats, helps stabilize blood sugar levels and provides sustained energy.
- Hydration: Dehydration can contribute to fatigue. Ensuring adequate water intake is vital for maintaining energy levels.

2. Inflammation and Pain Management:

- Anti-Inflammatory Foods: Some foods possess anti-inflammatory properties, which can be beneficial in managing fibromyalgia symptoms.
- Omega-3 Fatty Acids: Found in fatty fish, flaxseeds, and walnuts, omega-3s may help reduce inflammation and alleviate pain.

3. Mood and Mental Well-being:

- Serotonin-Boosting Foods: Certain foods, like those rich in tryptophan (found in turkey, nuts, and seeds), contribute to serotonin production. Serotonin is a neurotransmitter associated with mood regulation.
- Complex Carbohydrates: Foods like whole grains can help stabilize mood by promoting the production of serotonin.

4. Gut Health:

- Probiotics: Incorporating probiotic-rich foods, such as yogurt and fermented foods, supports a healthy gut. Gut health is increasingly recognized for its impact on overall well-being, including mental health.
- Fiber: Adequate fiber intake promotes digestive health and may alleviate symptoms related to irritable bowel syndrome (IBS), which is common in fibromyalgia.

5. Individualized Nutrition:

- Identifying Triggers: Paying attention to how your body responds to different foods helps identify potential triggers for symptoms.

- Consulting Professionals: Working with healthcare providers, including dietitians, can provide personalized dietary recommendations based on your unique needs.

6. Weight Management:

- Balanced Approach: Maintaining a healthy weight through a balanced and nutritious diet is important for overall health.
- Physical Activity: Combining proper nutrition with gentle physical activity supports weight management and enhances well-being.

7. Adequate Nutrient Intake:

- Vitamins and Minerals: Ensuring sufficient intake of vitamins and minerals, such as vitamin D and magnesium, is crucial for overall health and can contribute to symptom management.

8. Hydration and Medication Interaction:

- Medication Considerations: Some medications may impact nutrient absorption or interact with certain foods. Being mindful of these considerations is important.

- Hydration Impact: Proper hydration supports bodily functions and can influence how medications are metabolized.

Understanding the interconnected nature of nutrition and fibromyalgia empowers you to make informed choices that positively impact your energy levels and overall health. Regular communication with your healthcare team and incorporating a balanced, individualized approach to nutrition are key components of managing fibromyalgia effectively.

Incorporating Mindful Eating into Daily Life

Incorporating mindful eating into your daily life as a fibromyalgia patient can be a transformative journey, enhancing your relationship with food and supporting your overall well-being. Let's explore practical ways to integrate mindful eating practices, along with chair yoga exercises tailored for individuals with fibromyalgia:

Mindful Eating Strategies:

1. Create a Calm Eating Environment:

- Find a quiet and comfortable space for meals.
- Minimize distractions, such as electronic devices or television, to focus on your eating experience.

2. Engage Your Senses:

- Before taking a bite, observe the colors, textures, and aromas of your food.
- Pay attention to the act of chewing and savor the flavors.

3. Chew Slowly and Deliberately:

- Take your time with each bite, savoring the taste and texture.

- Aim for a slower pace to allow your body to signal fullness.

4. **Practice Gratitude:**

- Before starting your meal, take a moment to express gratitude for the nourishment in front of you.
- Cultivate a positive mindset around the act of eating.

5. **Listen to Your Body:**

- Tune in to your body's hunger and fullness cues.
- Eat when you're hungry and stop when you're satisfied.

6. **Mindful Portion Control:**

- Be aware of portion sizes, and avoid overloading your plate.
- Consider using smaller plates to help with portion control.

7. **Stay Hydrated:**

- Drink water throughout your meal to stay hydrated.

- Sipping water can also provide a moment of pause between bites.

8. **Mindful Snacking:**

- When snacking, choose nutrient-dense options.
- Pay attention to the experience of snacking rather than mindlessly consuming.

9. **Practice Mindful Breathing:**

- Take a few deep breaths before starting your meal to center yourself.
- Mindful breathing can help create a sense of calm.

Chair yoga practices that promote mindful eating.

1. **Seated Mountain Pose:**

- Sit comfortably in your chair, grounding your feet.

- Inhale, reaching your arms overhead, and exhale with awareness. This promotes a sense of presence.

2. **Seated Forward Bend:**

- Sit forward in your chair with feet flat on the floor.
- As you inhale, lengthen your spine, and as you exhale, hinge at your hips, reaching towards your toes. This fosters a connection between breath and movement.

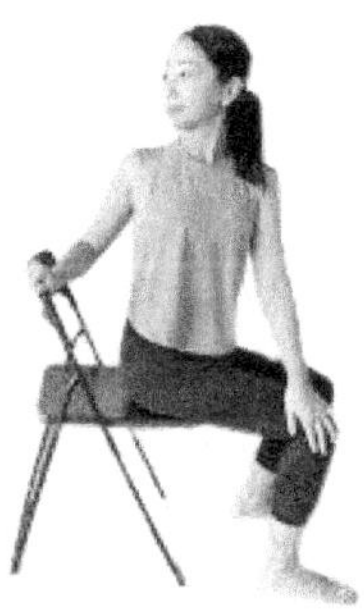

3. **Seated Spinal Twist:**

- Sit with a tall spine and twist gently to one side, holding the back of the chair for support.
- This twist promotes digestion and encourages mindful awareness of your body.

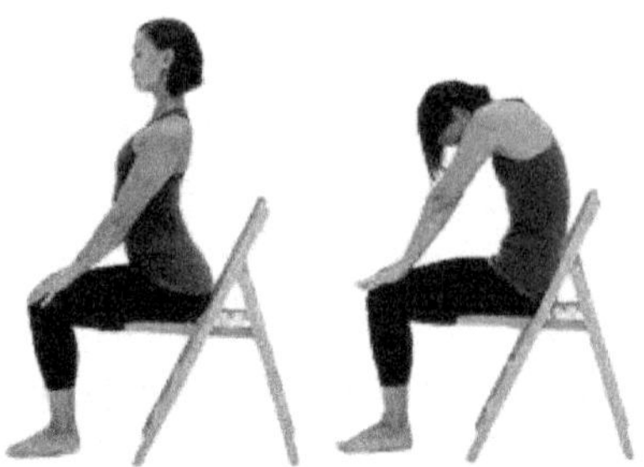

4. **Chair Cat-Cow Stretch:**

- Sit forward in your chair, place your hands on your knees.
- Inhale arching your back (Cow), and exhale rounding your spine (Cat). Coordinate this movement with your breath.

5. **Seated Tree Pose:**

- Ground one foot firmly on the floor and place the sole of the other foot against the inner thigh or calf.
- Focus on your breath and the connection between your body and the chair.

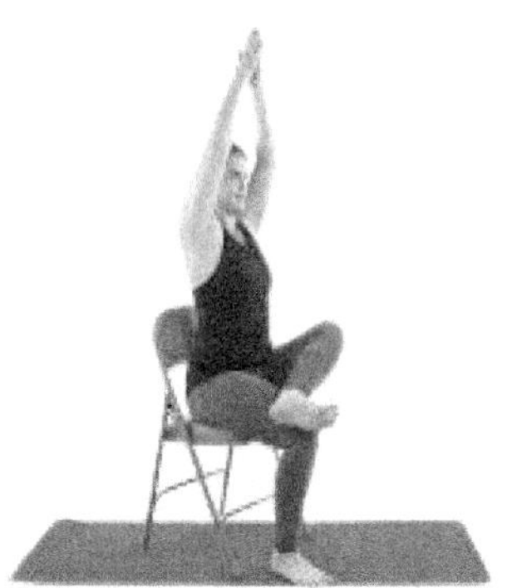

Combining mindful eating practices with these chair yoga exercises can create a holistic approach to nourishing your body and mind. Remember, the key is to approach each practice with gentleness and self-compassion, allowing these mindful moments to enhance your overall well-being as you navigate fibromyalgia.

14 Tips for creating a mindful eating environment.

Creating a mindful eating environment is an essential component of fostering a positive relationship with food, especially for individuals managing conditions like fibromyalgia.

Here are some practical tips tailored to your needs as a fibromyalgia patient:

1. Comfortable Seating:

- Choose a chair that provides ample support and comfort during meals.
- Consider using cushions or pillows for additional comfort, especially if you experience pain or discomfort while sitting.

2. Soft Lighting:

- Opt for soft, gentle lighting in your eating space.
- Harsh lighting can contribute to sensory overload, so adjusting the lighting to a calming level can enhance your dining experience.

3. Tranquil Atmosphere:

- Create a serene atmosphere by minimizing noise and distractions.
- Play soft, soothing music or enjoy your meal in quiet to promote a calm and relaxed environment.

4. Mindful Table Setting:

- Keep your dining area clutter-free and organized.
- Use simple and aesthetically pleasing tableware to enhance the visual appeal of your meal.

5. Engaging Senses:

- Incorporate elements that engage your senses positively.
- Use scented candles or fresh flowers to add a pleasant aroma to the environment.

6. Mindful Breathing Space:

- Set aside a few moments for mindful breathing before starting your meal.
- Practice deep, slow breaths to create a sense of calmness and presence.

7. Thoughtful Meal Planning:

- Plan meals that are both nourishing and enjoyable.

- Consider incorporating a variety of colors, textures, and flavors to make your meals visually appealing and satisfying.

8. Mindful Portion Control:

- Be mindful of portion sizes to prevent overeating.
- Consider using smaller plates and bowls to naturally control portion sizes.

9. Intuitive Eating Focus:

- Embrace intuitive eating by listening to your body's hunger and fullness cues.
- Avoid strict diet rules and instead, focus on eating with awareness and enjoyment.

10. Adaptive Seating Options:

- If sitting for extended periods is challenging, consider incorporating adaptive seating options.
- Use a comfortable cushion or consider a chair with additional support.

11. Hydration Station:

- Keep a water bottle within reach to stay hydrated.
- Staying hydrated supports overall well-being and can enhance the enjoyment of your meals.

12. Gentle Mealtime Rituals:

- Establish gentle rituals around mealtimes.
- This could include taking a moment to express gratitude or simply pausing before and after your meal to savor the experience.

13. Flexible Meal Timing:

- Allow flexibility in meal timing to accommodate your energy levels and daily schedule.
- Listen to your body and choose meal times that align with your natural rhythm.

14. Mindful Clean-Up:

- Extend mindfulness to the clean-up process.
- Wash dishes or tidy up mindfully, using the activity as a continuation of your mindful eating practice.

Remember, the goal is to create an environment that promotes a positive and mindful relationship with food, taking into consideration the unique challenges and sensitivities associated with fibromyalgia.

Balancing Nutrition and Movement

The relationship between activity and diet is critical to achieving comprehensive well-being.

An important factor in controlling weight is nutrition. A healthy weight may be maintained, and a proper dietary balance supports metabolic health.

Through mindful eating practices, individuals can become attuned to their body's hunger and fullness cues, fostering a sustainable approach to weight management.

Adequate nutrition is essential for muscle repair and growth, key components of strength-building. Nutrient-dense foods provide the energy needed for chair yoga sessions, enhancing overall performance and facilitating muscle recovery.

Chair yoga and mindful eating share common principles of mindfulness and awareness. Engaging in chair yoga with a focus on breath and movement heightens awareness, making individuals more attuned to their body's needs, including nutritional requirements.

A diet that is well-balanced and includes enough protein, healthy fats, and carbs will help you achieve your goals of gaining strength and managing your weight. Chair yoga sessions can be complemented by a pre-session snack or post-session meal, providing the necessary fuel for optimal performance and recovery.

Drinking enough water promotes general health and helps the body function properly during chair yoga sessions. Proper hydration aids digestion nutrient absorption, and helps prevent fatigue, contributing to an effective and enjoyable practice.

For example, meet Jessica, a determined individual on her journey to improved well-being. Struggling with weight management and seeking strength-building solutions,

Jessica discovered the transformative synergy of chair yoga and mindful eating.

By integrating chair yoga into her daily routine and adopting mindful eating practices, Jessica experienced positive changes in her body and mindset. The gentle movements of chair yoga complimented her weight management goals, while mindful eating allowed her to savour and appreciate the nourishment her body received.

Jessica's narrative underscores the potential for transformative change when nutrition and movement align harmoniously. Her narrative offers hope to anyone looking for a sustainable and well-rounded approach to well-being.

Balancing nutrition and movement is a dynamic process that can yield profound benefits for weight management and strength-building. By embracing mindful eating practices alongside chair yoga, you can create a symbiotic relationship that nourishes both body and mind, fostering positive changes and contributing to an overall sense of well-being.

Living with fibromyalgia presents unique challenges, and finding an exercise routine that accommodates your specific needs is crucial. Personalized chair yoga routines offer a gentle yet effective way to promote physical well-being, manage symptoms, and enhance the overall quality of life for individuals with fibromyalgia. This is why the next chapter opens us up to personal chair yoga routines that you can incorporate and adopt.

CHAPTER 8

Community Support and Motivation

***"Alone we can do so little, together we can do so much." -* Helen Keller.**

In the intricate journey of navigating fibromyalgia through the practice of chair yoga, the power of community stands as a beacon of strength. Helen Keller's words echo profoundly, encapsulating the essence of finding resilience and encouragement not in solitude but within the embrace of a supportive community.

In the realm of fibromyalgia, where each day may present unique challenges, a community provides a sanctuary of shared understanding. Fellow practitioners comprehend the nuances of the condition, fostering empathy and camaraderie.

A community becomes a collective narrative of triumphs, both big and small. Witnessing others navigate and conquer similar obstacles becomes a wellspring of motivation, inspiring individuals to persist in their chair yoga practice.

Fibromyalgia, with its physical and emotional toll, necessitates a network of emotional support. A community serves as a virtual shoulder to lean on, offering encouragement during challenging times and celebrating victories together. Chair yoga communities tailor their support to the unique needs of individuals with fibromyalgia. The adaptability of chair yoga, coupled with a community's understanding, creates an inclusive space for all levels of ability.

Consistency in chair yoga practice is often challenging for those managing fibromyalgia symptoms. A supportive community provides the motivation needed to stay consistent, turning the practice into a communal journey.

Communities become a rich source of knowledge. Members share insights, tips, and modifications that have worked for them, enhancing the collective wisdom of the group and enriching each practitioner's experience.

As a fibromyalgia patient practicing chair yoga, the strength derived from a supportive community is immeasurable. It transforms the solitary path of managing a neurological condition into a shared odyssey, where challenges are faced collectively and victories are savored together. In the inspiring words of Helen Keller, the journey becomes a testament to the profound truth that in community, resilience is not just found—it flourishes, creating a tapestry of support, motivation, and shared strength.

The Role of Community in Neurological Well-being

The role of the community in promoting neurological well-being, particularly in the context of individuals dealing with Fibromyalgia, is profound and multifaceted. In this regard, the supportive network offered by a community becomes instrumental in managing both the physical and emotional aspects of the condition.

Emotional support is a cornerstone of community involvement for individuals grappling with Fibromyalgia. The nature of this condition often leads to feelings of isolation and frustration, as the symptoms can be challenging to understand for those who do not experience them firsthand. Connecting with a group of people who have gone through similar things as you do might make you feel validated and like you belong. It offers a forum where people may freely express their ideas and feelings without worrying about being judged, fostering an environment where they feel understood and encouraged.

The emotional support derived from the community plays a pivotal role in coping with the psychological impact of the condition. The shared experiences within the community not only validate the emotional struggles but also offer coping strategies and encouragement.

Moreover, the community serves as an invaluable source of information and resources. Fibromyalgia is a complex condition, and navigating its management can be overwhelming. A supportive community provides a platform for individuals to share insights into various treatments, coping mechanisms, and lifestyle adjustments that have proven effective in managing symptoms. People who are empowered to make educated decisions regarding their health and well-being can benefit from this knowledge sharing.

In addition to emotional support and information sharing, community involvement for Fibromyalgia patients can contribute to advocacy efforts. Raising awareness about the condition, dispelling myths, and promoting understanding within the broader community are essential components of advocacy. By working together, those who have Fibromyalgia may lessen the stigma attached to the illness and promote a more accepting and inclusive community.

The role of the community in the neurological well-being of Fibromyalgia patients cannot be overstated. Beyond emotional support, communities provide a vital platform for information exchange, coping strategies, and advocacy. These communities provide a substantial contribution to the overall well-being of those coping with the difficulties presented by Fibromyalgia by creating a sense of acceptance and understanding.

Creating or Joining Chair Yoga Communities

Establishing or becoming part of Chair Yoga communities, specifically tailored for individuals with Fibromyalgia like yourself, can be a powerful and enriching journey. These communities, whether online or offline, serve as valuable resources, offering both a means of engaging in gentle physical activity and connecting with others who understand the unique challenges posed by Fibromyalgia.

Creating Chair Yoga Communities:

- **Online Platforms:**

Social Media Groups: Explore and join Facebook or Reddit groups dedicated to Fibromyalgia, and consider creating a subgroup within these communities that focuses on Chair Yoga. This allows for more personalized discussions and the sharing of Chair Yoga resources.

Dedicated Forums: You may consider setting up an independent forum or website specifically for individuals with Fibromyalgia who are interested in Chair Yoga. This could serve as a centralized space for sharing experiences and accessing helpful information.

Local Meetups:

Community Centers and Libraries: Investigate the possibility of collaborating with local community centers or libraries to organize regular Chair Yoga sessions for individuals with Fibromyalgia. This can provide a physical space for community members to connect and support one another.

Wellness Events: Keep an eye out for or actively participate in wellness events focusing on Fibromyalgia and Chair Yoga. These events could include workshops, seminars, or health fairs.

Joining Chair Yoga Communities:

- **Online Resources:**

Yoga Apps and Websites: Explore yoga apps or websites that offer Chair Yoga classes specifically designed for individuals with chronic conditions such as Fibromyalgia. Platforms like Glo or Yoga for the Inflexible may provide suitable programs for practicing from the comfort of your home.

YouTube Channels: Subscribe to YouTube channels where instructors create content tailored to those with chronic pain conditions. This can be a convenient way to access guided Chair Yoga sessions.

- **Local Support Groups:**

Healthcare Facilities: Inquire at local hospitals, clinics, or rehabilitation centers about support groups or programs that integrate Chair Yoga for individuals with Fibromyalgia.

Community Centers: Check with community centers for wellness programs, including adaptive yoga classes. Bulletin boards or websites may have information about scheduled sessions.

- **Community Events:**

Health and Wellness Expos: Attend events that focus on health and wellness, where you may discover information about Chair Yoga classes specifically designed for individuals with chronic conditions.

Local Yoga Studios: Reach out to local yoga studios to inquire about specialized classes or workshops for those with chronic pain, like individuals with Fibromyalgia.

Whether you're starting these communities or already belong to one, the focus is on building a safe space where you can talk about your experiences, get advice from others, and have access to tools that improve your general health. This journey is about building a sense of community and empowerment as you navigate the unique aspects of Fibromyalgia.

Engaging in shared practice and receiving encouragement within a community setting can offer profound benefits for individuals managing Fibromyalgia. As someone navigating the challenges of Fibromyalgia, the support and camaraderie derived from shared practice and encouragement can positively impact various aspects of your well-being.

1. Mutual Understanding and Empathy:

Participating in a community of individuals with Fibromyalgia fosters a shared understanding of the condition. Others in the community have firsthand experience with the physical and emotional challenges you face, creating a supportive environment where empathy flourishes.

2. Emotional Support:

Fibromyalgia can be emotionally taxing, and the shared practice within a community provides a safe space to express your feelings. Help from others who are aware of the difficulties you are facing may be emotionally stimulating, reducing feelings of isolation and fostering a sense of belonging.

3. Motivation and Accountability:

The encouragement received from fellow community members can serve as a powerful motivator. Knowing that others are on a similar journey creates a sense of collective determination, inspiring you to stay committed to your well-being goals. The mutual encouragement within the community fosters a shared commitment to overcoming challenges.

4. Collective Learning and Resource Sharing:

Shared practice allows for the exchange of valuable insights and coping strategies. Other individuals with Fibromyalgia may offer practical tips and resources that have proven effective in managing symptoms.

This collaborative learning enhances your knowledge and empowers you to make informed decisions about your health.

5. Reduction of Stigma and Validation:

Encountering shared experiences within the community helps validate the reality of Fibromyalgia. As community members share their triumphs and struggles, it contributes to reducing the stigma associated with the condition. Feeling validated in your experiences promotes a sense of acceptance and understanding.

6. Social Connection and Sense of Belonging:

Fibromyalgia can lead to social isolation, but engaging in shared practice provides an avenue for social connection. Building relationships with others who share similar challenges creates a sense of belonging and community, positively impacting your mental and emotional well-being.

7. Enhanced Coping Mechanisms:

Encouragement from the community often involves sharing successful coping mechanisms and strategies.

Learning from others' experiences can broaden your toolkit for managing symptoms, enhancing your ability to navigate the complexities of Fibromyalgia more effectively.

8. Positive Impact on Mental Health:

The encouragement received within a supportive community contributes to positive mental health outcomes. Shared practice fosters a sense of hope and resilience, crucial elements in coping with the uncertainties and fluctuations associated with Fibromyalgia.

As a Fibromyalgia patient, engaging in shared practice and receiving encouragement within a community setting offers a range of benefits. From emotional support and motivation to collective learning and a sense of belonging, the positive impact of participating in a supportive community can significantly enhance your overall well-being.

Motivational Stories of Community Impact

Here are narratives of individuals who found inspiration and motivation within a chair yoga community, highlighting the transformative effect of community support on their adherence to the practice.

1. Susan's Journey to Renewed Strength:

Susan, a Fibromyalgia patient, discovered a chair yoga community online. Initially hesitant due to her physical limitations, Susan found inspiration in the stories of others who had experienced similar challenges. Through the community's encouragement and shared experiences, Susan gradually embraced chair yoga. Over time, she not only improved her physical strength but also found a renewed sense of empowerment and motivation to continue her practice.

2. John's Resilience in the Face of Chronic Pain:

Dealing with chronic pain from Fibromyalgia, John joined a local chair yoga group organized by a community center. The supportive atmosphere and the camaraderie with fellow participants became a source of motivation for John. As he witnessed the progress of others facing similar struggles, he felt inspired to persevere despite his pain. The community's positive impact fueled John's determination, leading to increased adherence to his chair yoga practice and noticeable improvements in his overall well being.

3. Maria's Emotional Healing Through Connection:

Maria, facing the emotional toll of Fibromyalgia, joined an online chair yoga community. She made connections with others who shared the emotional as well as the physical difficulties of dealing with chronic pain through online discussions. The mutual encouragement and understanding provided Maria with a sense of emotional healing. The community support became a driving force, motivating her to maintain a consistent chair yoga practice as a means of holistic well-being.

4. Robert's Journey to Stress Reduction:

Robert, managing Fibromyalgia-related stress, became part of a chair yoga community at his local wellness center. The practice not only alleviated his physical discomfort but also became a crucial tool for stress reduction. The encouragement from the community members, who shared their own stories of stress relief through chair yoga, inspired Robert to integrate the practice into his daily routine. The positive impact on his mental health reinforced his commitment to the community and the chair yoga practice.

5. Emily's Empowerment Through Shared Success:

Emily, a Fibromyalgia patient navigating mobility challenges, found empowerment in a chair yoga community that celebrated shared successes. Witnessing others overcoming obstacles and achieving milestones fueled Emily's determination. The community's emphasis on celebrating each participant's progress, no matter how small, instilled a sense of achievement in Emily. This collective encouragement became a driving force in her commitment to chair yoga as a transformative aspect of her wellness journey.

The positive impact of community support on adherence to chair yoga practice

The positive impact of community support on adherence to chair yoga practice for individuals coping with Fibromyalgia is a testament to the transformative influence that a supportive community can have on overall well-being. Chronic pain and exhaustion are the hallmarks of fibromyalgia, which poses special difficulties that can frequently result in physical limits and feelings of loneliness. Engaging in chair yoga within a supportive community setting provides a range of benefits that significantly enhance adherence to the practice.

1. Emotional Support and Understanding:

For people with Fibromyalgia, the emotional support provided by a chair yoga group is priceless. A sense of connection and understanding is fostered by sharing experiences, difficulties, and victories with others who are aware of the obstacles people face on a daily basis. This emotional support acts as a motivational factor, encouraging individuals to stay committed to their chair yoga practice.

2. Motivation Through Shared Success Stories:

Witnessing the positive outcomes and success stories of fellow community members who have experienced improvements in their well-being through chair yoga serves as powerful motivation. These shared successes inspire individuals to believe in the effectiveness of the practice and fuel their commitment to incorporating it into their routine.

3. Collective Accountability:

Being part of a chair yoga community creates a sense of collective accountability. People are more likely to stick with a practice they are devoted to when they know that others have similar objectives. The mutual encouragement within the community establishes a supportive environment where members hold each other accountable, contributing to sustained adherence.

4. Practical Tips and Advice:

Community support facilitates the exchange of practical tips and advice on integrating chair yoga into daily life. Fibromyalgia patients often face unique challenges, and the community becomes a valuable resource for discovering adaptations and modifications that make the practice more accessible. This shared knowledge enhances the overall experience and encourages continued engagement.

5. Reduction of Isolation and Stigma:

Fibromyalgia can lead to feelings of isolation and a sense of being misunderstood. Being part of a chair yoga community counters this isolation by fostering a sense of belonging. The collective understanding within the community reduces the stigma associated with chronic pain conditions, creating a positive environment that encourages regular participation.

6. Sense of Community and Belonging:

Establishing a sense of community and belonging is crucial for Fibromyalgia patients. The support and encouragement from fellow community members create a positive and inclusive atmosphere. This sense of community becomes a motivating factor as individuals feel a shared commitment to their well-being through the practice of chair yoga.

7. Continuous Learning and Adaptation:

Through the community, people may continually modify their chair yoga practice based on shared experiences, creating a dynamic learning environment. This adaptive approach ensures that the practice remains tailored to the unique needs of Fibromyalgia patients, enhancing its effectiveness and promoting sustained adherence.

CHAPTER 9

Personalized Chair Yoga Routines

The positive impact of community support on adherence to chair yoga practice for Fibromyalgia patients extends beyond the physical benefits of the practice. Emotional support, shared successes, and the sense of belonging within a community contribute significantly to a supportive environment that empowers individuals to stay committed to their chair yoga journey, ultimately enhancing their overall well-being.

Assessing personal health goals and challenges.

Setting off on a path of self-awareness and wellness necessitates carefully considering your health objectives as well as the difficulties brought on by fibromyalgia. By recognizing and understanding your needs, you lay the foundation for a chair yoga practice that aligns seamlessly with your journey.

1. Identifying Health Goals:

Take a moment to reflect on your overarching health objectives. Whether it's managing pain, improving flexibility, enhancing mood, or fostering relaxation, clearly defining your goals provides a roadmap for your chair yoga practice. Your goals serve as guiding stars, steering your practice toward tangible and meaningful outcomes.

2. Acknowledging Challenges:

Fibromyalgia presents a spectrum of challenges, both physical and emotional. Identify and acknowledge these challenges with honesty and compassion. Whether it's coping with chronic pain, managing fatigue, or navigating stress, recognizing the obstacles you face allows for a targeted and empathetic approach in tailoring your chair yoga routine.

3. Establishing Realistic Expectations:

For your chair yoga practice, set reasonable goals that correspond to your present state of energy and ability. Embrace the concept of gradual Progress and listen to your body's cues. Understanding that each session may differ allows you to approach your practice with flexibility and adaptability.

4. Crafting a Personalized Routine:

Armed with insights into your health goals and challenges, work towards crafting a personalized chair yoga routine. Tailor your practice to address specific areas of concern, incorporating poses and sequences that resonate with your objectives. In addition to increasing the practice's efficacy, this individualized approach gives you a greater sense of control over your health.

5. Seeking Professional Guidance:

Consider consulting with healthcare professionals or certified yoga instructors experienced in working with Fibromyalgia patients. Their knowledge may offer insightful information that will guarantee your chair yoga practice is secure, efficient, and tailored to your particular requirements.

6. Embracing Mind-Body Connection:

Recognize the interconnectedness of mind and body. Your chair yoga practice is an opportunity to cultivate a harmonious relationship between the two. Use breathwork and mindfulness to help you de-stress, become more at ease, and feel better all around.

7. Celebrating Progress:

Celebrate the small victories along your journey. Whether it's increased flexibility, improved mood, or a sense of calm, acknowledging and celebrating Progress reinforces a positive mindset. Your chair yoga practice becomes a continuous celebration of your resilience and commitment to self-care.

In understanding your needs as a Fibromyalgia patient and assessing personal health goals and challenges, you lay the groundwork for a chair yoga practice that is not only tailored to your unique circumstances but also empowers you to take active ownership of your well-being. This self-directed approach fosters a sense of agency, resilience, and a deeper connection to the transformative potential of chair yoga in your life.

Neurological conditions such as Fibromyalgia often necessitate individualized approaches to address the diverse and complex nature of symptoms and challenges associated with these conditions. Recognizing the unique characteristics of each person's experience becomes paramount in developing effective strategies for management and improvement.

Due to the variability of symptoms and their intensity among individuals with Fibromyalgia, an individualized treatment plan is crucial. In order to tailor treatments that address certain symptoms, medical practitioners can collaborate with patients and take into account variables, including pain intensity, weariness, and emotional stability.

Physical activity, including chair yoga, plays a significant role in managing Fibromyalgia symptoms. Recognizing that each person may have distinct physical limitations, preferences, and goals, healthcare providers can recommend personalized exercise regimens. This approach ensures that the chosen exercises address the individual's unique needs without exacerbating symptoms.

Medication management for Fibromyalgia varies from person to person. Individualized approaches involve carefully selecting and adjusting medications based on the specific symptoms and response to treatment. This personalized medication strategy aims to optimize efficacy while minimizing side effects.

Cognitive and behavioral therapies are essential components of Fibromyalgia management. Tailoring these therapies to address individual psychological and emotional aspects ensures a more comprehensive approach. Addressing specific challenges such as stress, anxiety, and sleep disturbances can contribute to an improved quality of life.

Their diet and way of living can greatly impact fibromyalgia sufferers' well-being. Recognizing the unique dietary needs and lifestyle considerations of each person allows for personalized guidance. This may include recommendations for anti-inflammatory diets, stress management techniques, and sleep hygiene practices tailored to individual preferences and circumstances.

Psychosocial support is crucial in addressing the emotional toll of Fibromyalgia. Individualized counseling and support groups provide a space for patients to discuss their unique challenges, coping mechanisms, and emotional well-being.

Recognizing the individual nature of these experiences fosters a more supportive and empathetic environment.

Given the dynamic nature of Fibromyalgia symptoms, individualized approaches involve regular monitoring and adjustments to treatment plans. To guarantee continued efficacy, healthcare professionals can collaborate closely with patients to monitor development, reevaluate objectives, and adjust interventions as necessary.

Acknowledging the need for individualized approaches in managing neurological conditions like Fibromyalgia is essential for optimizing care and improving overall outcomes.

Adapting Chair Yoga Poses for Personalization

Adapting chair yoga poses to suit individual requirements is a crucial aspect of personalization, especially for individuals managing conditions like Fibromyalgia. Here's a guide on how to modify chair yoga poses based on your unique needs:

1. Seated Mountain Pose (Tadasana):

Modification:

- Sit comfortably in the chair with your feet flat. Feel free to adjust the distance between your feet based on your comfort.
- Ground your sit bones into the chair, lengthen your spine, and lift your chest.
- This modification maintains the essence of the pose while accommodating your requirements.

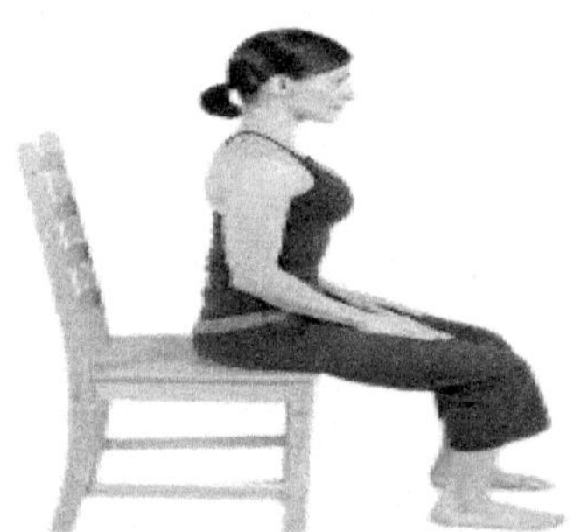

2. Seated Forward Bend (Paschimottanasana):

Modification:

- Sit at the edge of the chair with your feet flat on the ground.
- Hinge at your hips, leading with your chest, and gently fold forward.
- Allow your hands to reach towards your feet or the floor. This modification minimizes strain on the lower back and adapts the pose to your comfort level.

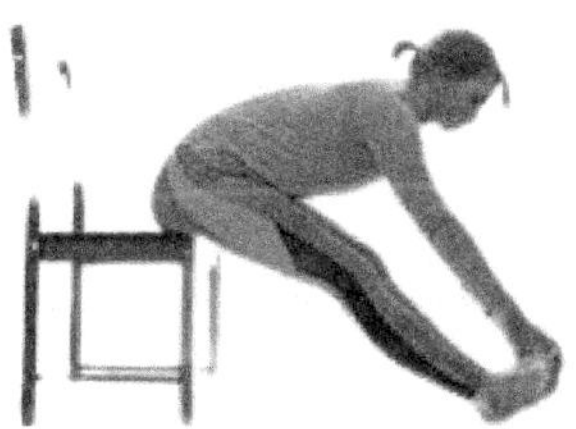

3. Seated Cat-Cow Stretch:

Modification:

- Take an upright position on the chair with your hands on your knees.
- Breathe in, raising your chest and arching your back (Cow Pose).

- Exhale, rounding your spine and bringing your chin to your chest (Cat Pose).
- This seated variation helps spinal mobility without putting pressure on the wrists or knees.

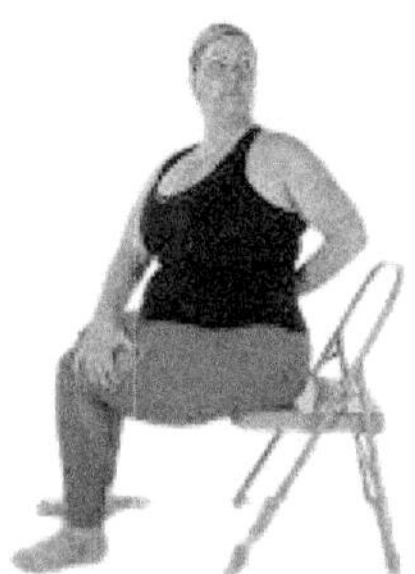

4. Seated Twist (Ardha Matsyendrasana):

Modification:

- Sit comfortably in the chair, placing one hand on the opposite knee and the other on the back.
- Gently twist your torso, looking over your shoulder.
- This modification ensures a gentle stretch through the spine and avoids excessive twisting for those with Fibromyalgia.

5. Seated Warrior Pose:

Modification:

- Sit with your feet planted firmly on the ground.
- Extend one leg forward and bend the opposite knee, placing the foot on the inner thigh.
- Raise your arms overhead, palms facing each other.
- This modification provides a grounding stretch without the need to stand.

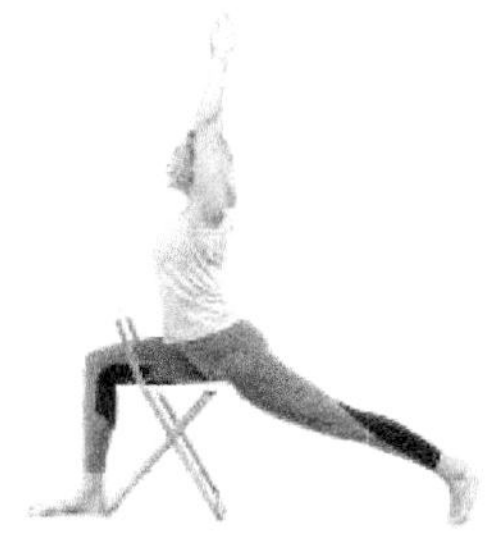

6. Chair Pigeon Pose:

Modification:

- Sit on the edge of the chair, cross one ankle over the opposite knee, and gently press down on the lifted knee.
- This adapted Pigeon Pose helps release hip tension without requiring you to come to the floor.

7. Chair Warrior II Pose:

Modification:

- Sit with your feet wide apart, toes pointing slightly outward.
- Rotate your upper body towards one side, bringing one arm forward and the other back.
- This modification allows you to experience the essence of Warrior II while seated.

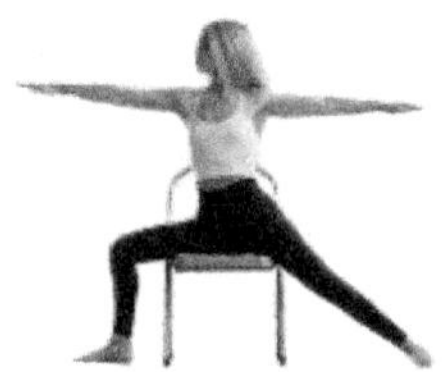

8. Seated Tree Pose:

Modification:

- Comfortably sit with one foot's sole resting on the calf or inner thigh of the other leg.
- Grasp the chair for stability. This adjustment offers a little stretch to the thighs and hips while preserving strength and balance.
- This modification maintains balance and stability while providing a gentle hip and thigh stretch.

9. Gentle Neck Stretches:

Modification:

- As you sit up straight, turn your head slightly to the side and place your ear on your shoulder.
- Change sides after a few breaths of holding.
- This modified neck stretch helps release tension without the need for complicated movements.

10. Savasana (Relaxation Pose):

Modification:

- Sit comfortably in the chair, close your eyes, and focus on your breath.
- Allow your body to relax in the chair.
- This adapted Savasana provides a refreshing experience without lying on the floor.

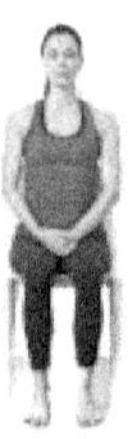

Remember, the key is to listen to your body and make modifications that suit your comfort and well-being. Feel free to adapt poses as needed, emphasizing gentle movements and comfort to make your chair yoga practice accessible and enjoyable.

Incorporating variety to maintain interest and motivation.

Maintaining interest and motivation in your chair yoga practice as a Fibromyalgia patient is essential for long-term engagement and overall well-being. Adding variation to your routine will assist in maintaining the sustainability, enjoyment, and freshness of your practice.

Here are some strategies to introduce diversity to your chair yoga sessions:

1. Explore Different Styles of Chair Yoga:

Experiment with various styles of chair yoga. From gentle and restorative sessions to more dynamic practices, each class offers a unique experience. You can find the strategy that best suits your requirements and tastes by experimenting with numerous techniques.

2. Rotate Focus Areas:

Vary the focus of your chair yoga practice. For instance, dedicate sessions to flexibility, balance, or relaxation. By rotating emphasis on different aspects of well-being, you keep your routine interesting while addressing specific needs in each session.

3. Add New Poses Gradually:

Introduce new chair yoga poses gradually to prevent monotony. Include one or two new poses per session, allowing time to become familiar with each movement. This approach maintains interest and provides a sense of accomplishment as you expand your repertoire.

4. Modify Sequences:

Modify your chair yoga sequences regularly. Change the order of poses or explore different combinations to create a fresh experience. Modifying sequences challenges your body in new ways and prevents the routine from becoming predictable.

5. Utilize Props and Accessories:

Incorporate props and accessories into your chair yoga practice. Small props like resistance bands, cushions, or yoga blocks can add variety and enhance the effectiveness of specific exercises. These tools provide new dimensions to your practice and make it more engaging.

6. Combine Chair Yoga with Other Activities:

Integrate chair yoga with other activities you enjoy. For example, listen to calming music, nature sounds, or a guided meditation during practice. Combining chair yoga with enjoyable elements enhances the overall experience and makes it a more pleasant routine.

7. Attend Chair Yoga Classes or Workshops:

Attend chair yoga classes or workshops, either in-person or online. Participating in guided sessions led by an instructor introduces diversity and can expose you to different teaching styles and techniques. The communal aspect of group classes can also provide motivation and a sense of community.

8. Set Personal Challenges:

Challenge yourself by setting personal goals. Whether holding a pose for a longer duration or gradually increasing the intensity of specific movements, unique challenges add an element of excitement and achievement to your chair yoga practice.

9. Alternate with Other Forms of Exercise:

Alternate chair yoga with other forms of exercise that align with your abilities and preferences. This could include gentle walks, swimming, or seated strength training. Combining various activities ensures a holistic approach to your overall well-being.

10. Prioritize Enjoyment and Mindfulness:

Prioritize enjoyment and mindfulness in your chair yoga practice. Please focus on the pleasure of movement, the calming effect of your breath, and the sense of well-being it brings. A mindful and enjoyable practice is more likely to be sustained over time.

By embracing variety in your chair yoga routine, you enhance its physical benefits and contribute to sustained interest and motivation. Remember, the key is to create a practice that aligns with your preferences, adapts to your needs, and remains an enjoyable and fulfilling part of your well-being journey as a Fibromyalgia patient.

Incorporating Mindfulness in Personalized Practice

Incorporating mindfulness into your personalized chair yoga practice as a Fibromyalgia patient is a powerful approach to enhancing your mental and physical well-being. Mindfulness plays a crucial role in adapting chair yoga to your needs by fostering a heightened awareness of your body, breathing, and the present moment.

Here's how you can integrate mindfulness into your practice:

1. Mindful Breath Awareness:

Begin your chair yoga session by bringing attention to your breath. Mindful breathing involves observing each inhalation and exhalation. As a Fibromyalgia patient, focusing on your breath creates a calming anchor and promotes relaxation, reducing stress that may exacerbate symptoms.

2. Gentle Body Scans:

Incorporate gentle body scans throughout your practice. Mindfully direct your awareness to different body parts, noting sensations, tension, or comfort areas. This self-awareness allows you to adapt chair yoga poses based on real-time feedback from your body.

3. Mindful Movement Transitions:

Approach each movement with mindfulness. Whether transitioning between chair yoga poses or adjusting your posture, be fully present in the action. Mindful transitions enhance body awareness, reduce the risk of overexertion, and allow for a more fluid and comfortable practice.

4. Cultivate Non-Judgmental Awareness:

Practice non-judgmental awareness of your thoughts and sensations. If discomfort arises during a pose, approach it without judgment. Acknowledge the feelings without labeling them as good or bad. This non-judgmental attitude fosters self-compassion and reduces stress associated with physical challenges.

5. Mindful Alignment and Modification:

Pay attention to the alignment of your body in each chair yoga pose. Mindfully adjust your position to find a comfortable and sustainable alignment. Mindful modification is about adapting poses to suit your unique needs, ensuring you experience the benefits without strain.

6. Present-Moment Awareness:

Embrace present-moment awareness in your chair yoga practice. Allow your attention to reside in the current moment rather than dwelling on past experiences or anticipating future challenges. Mindful presence enhances the therapeutic aspects of chair yoga and contributes to a positive mental outlook.

7. Use Guided Mindfulness Meditation:

Integrate guided mindfulness meditation into your practice. This could involve seated meditation at the beginning or end of your chair yoga session. Guided mindfulness helps cultivate a focused and calm mind, contributing to overall well-being.

8. Mindful Gratitude Practice:

Conclude your chair yoga practice with a mindful gratitude practice. Reflect on aspects of your body, mind, or life you are grateful for. Cultivating gratitude enhances the positive aspects of your experience, promoting a sense of contentment and satisfaction.

9. Mindful Relaxation Techniques:

Explore mindful relaxation techniques, such as progressive muscle relaxation or guided imagery, to enhance the relaxation benefits of chair yoga.

10. Regular Mindfulness Check-Ins:

Throughout your chair yoga practice, conduct regular mindfulness check-ins. Pause and tune into your breath, body sensations, and emotional state. These brief moments of mindfulness create a continuous thread of awareness, anchoring you in the present and optimizing the benefits of your practice.

By infusing mindfulness into your chair yoga practice, you create a holistic and adaptive approach that aligns with your individual needs as a Fibromyalgia patient.

Creating a sustainable and enjoyable routine.

Creating a sustainable and enjoyable routine as a Fibromyalgia patient requires a thoughtful and adaptive approach that considers your unique needs and challenges. Here's a guide to help you establish a way that promotes well-being while accommodating the specific requirements associated with Fibromyalgia:

- **Set Realistic Goals:**

Set attainable and reasonable goals at the outset of your routine. Break down your objectives into manageable steps, acknowledging the fluctuating nature of Fibromyalgia symptoms. Realistic goals provide a sense of accomplishment and motivation.

- **Prioritize Consistency Over Intensity:**

Emphasize consistency in your routine rather than pushing for intensity. Regular, moderate activity is often more beneficial than sporadic, intense sessions. The surface helps your body adapt and reduces the risk of exacerbating symptoms.

- **Choose Enjoyable Activities:**

Incorporate activities that you genuinely enjoy. Whether it's chair yoga, gentle stretching, or activities outside of exercise, selecting enjoyable pursuits increases motivation and makes your routine more sustainable.

- **Build Gradually:**

Build your routine gradually to avoid overexertion. Start with shorter sessions and slowly increase duration or intensity as your body adapts. This gradual approach minimizes the risk of symptom flare-ups and supports long-term sustainability.

- **Include Variety:**

Introduce Variety into your routine to keep it interesting. This can involve rotating between different exercises and activities or incorporating elements like mindfulness or relaxation techniques. Variety not only adds enjoyment but also prevents monotony.

- **Listen to Your Body:**

During and after each exercise, pay special attention to the signals coming from your body. If a particular activity or routine causes discomfort, adjust or modify it to better suit your needs. Listening to your body promotes a safer and more sustainable approach.

- **Establish a Consistent Schedule:**

Set a consistent schedule for your routine. Having practice helps your body anticipate and adapt to activity patterns. Consistency in timing also aids in forming a healthy habit that becomes more ingrained over time.

- **Prioritize Rest and Recovery:**

Acknowledge the significance of healing and relaxation in your daily regimen. Allow time for your body to recuperate after activities, and ensure that your training includes ample rest periods. Balancing activity with sufficient rest is crucial for managing Fibromyalgia symptoms.

- **Adapt Activities to Your Energy Levels:**

Align your routine with your energy levels. Schedule activities when you feel more energetic, and avoid pushing yourself during fatigue. This adaptive approach ensures your training is tailored to your body's natural rhythms.

- **Seek Support and Accountability:**

Engage the support of friends, family, or a healthcare professional to help you stay accountable to your routine. A support system provides encouragement, understanding, and motivation, making it easier to adhere to your plan.

- **Prioritize Self-Care:**

Integrate self-care practices into your routine. This can include warm baths, gentle massages, or mindfulness exercises. Prioritizing self-care contributes to overall well-being and enhances the sustainability of your way.

- **Celebrate Achievements:**

Celebrate both minor and significant achievements in your routine. Recognizing your progress, no matter how incremental reinforces a positive mindset and motivates continued engagement.

By tailoring your routine to prioritize enjoyment, consistency, and adaptability, you create a sustainable and enjoyable approach to managing Fibromyalgia. This personalized routine becomes a valuable tool in enhancing your overall well-being while accommodating the unique challenges associated with your condition.

Just before we draw the curtain on this chapter, let me quickly tell you a short story. In the small town of Harmonyville, a Fibromyalgia patient, Emily, discovered the transformative power of personalized chair yoga routines. Her journey, marked by pain and uncertainty, took an uplifting turn when she committed to tailoring her practice to align with her individual needs.

Emily's personalized chair yoga journey began with carefully considering her symptoms and limitations. Recognizing the importance of gentleness and adaptability, she crafted a routine that incorporated a variety of seated poses, mindful breathing exercises, and gentle stretches.

Emily faced moments of doubt and frustration as she embarked on this journey. However, guided by self-awareness and self-compassion, she learned to adapt her practice to accommodate fluctuations in her energy levels and pain thresholds. Each modification, whether a gentle twist or a modified forward bend, reflected Emily's commitment to making her chair yoga routine her own.

Over time, Emily witnessed remarkable improvements in her well-being. The gentle movements increased her flexibility, and the mindful breathing techniques became a source of solace during challenging moments. Most importantly, the personalized nature of her routine provided a sense of control and empowerment over her Fibromyalgia journey.

As the pages of Emily's story unfold, we are reminded of the profound impact personalized chair yoga can have on individuals facing Fibromyalgia. Her experience inspires fellow patients, encouraging them to embrace the uniqueness of their journeys.

Your Fibromyalgia journey is uniquely yours, and within the realm of personalized chair yoga lies the potential for profound transformation. Experiment with adaptations, modify poses to suit your comfort, and celebrate the victories, no matter how small.

As Emily found strength in customizing her chair yoga routine, you can also discover resilience, empowerment, and a renewed sense of well-being. Embrace the personalized approach to chair yoga, and may it become a valuable companion in your pursuit of comfort, strength, and joy on your Fibromyalgia journey.

CHAPTER 10

THE 30-DAY CHAIR YOGA CHALLENGE

"In the face of challenge, we discover our true strength and the transformative power within us."

In the heart of your Fibromyalgia journey, where resilience meets opportunity, we embark on a transformative odyssey—a 30-day Chair Yoga Challenge explicitly designed for you. Challenges are not merely obstacles; they are gateways to growth, and within this journey lies the potential for profound healing and well-being.

As a Fibromyalgia patient, the prospect of a 30-day challenge may seem both exhilarating and daunting. However, within the embrace of this challenge, you will discover the remarkable capacity of chair yoga to adapt, uplift, and empower.

Embarking on a journey towards well-being requires both commitment and adaptability, especially when navigating the unique challenges of Fibromyalgia. I invite you to embark on a transformative 30-day Chair Yoga Challenge—an empowering expedition to nurture your body, mind, and spirit.

This structured challenge is crafted with the understanding that each day presents a new opportunity for growth and self-discovery. With its gentle movements and mindful approach, chair yoga is a powerful tool for enhancing flexibility, managing pain, and fostering a deeper connection to your body.

Critical Elements of the 30-Day Challenge:

1. Daily Personalization:

Tailor each day's chair yoga routine to align with your individual needs. Whether you are focusing on specific muscle groups, relaxation, or gentle stretching, the emphasis is on personalization to accommodate the dynamic nature of Fibromyalgia.

2. Mindful Awareness:

Cultivate mindful awareness throughout the challenge. Pay attention to your body's signals, breath, and sensations. Mindfulness enhances the therapeutic benefits of chair yoga and contributes to a greater sense of self-awareness.

3. Gradual Progression:

Embrace a gradual progression in intensity and duration. Start with shorter sessions and allow your body to adapt over time. The goal is to build a sustainable and enjoyable routine supporting your well-being.

4. Weekly Themes:

Each week will have a thematic focus, incorporating a variety of poses and practices. Themes may include flexibility, strength, balance, relaxation, and mindfulness. This structure adds variety to your routine and addresses different aspects of your well-being.

5. Community Support:

Connect with a supportive community of participants. Share your experiences, challenges, and triumphs in a dedicated online space where you can connect with like-minded people and receive support. The community provides encouragement, understanding, and shared strength throughout the 30-day journey.

6. Weekly Reflections:

Engage in weekly reflections to assess your progress, both physically and emotionally. Reflecting on your experiences allows you to celebrate achievements, identify areas for growth, and deepen your connection to the transformative power of chair yoga.

7. Self-Care Integration:

Integrate self-care practices beyond the chair yoga sessions. Explore additional activities that promote relaxation, such as warm baths, gentle massages, or moments of mindful reflection. Holistic self-care contributes to a more comprehensive well-being strategy.

8. Celebrate Milestones:

Celebrate milestones along the way. Whether completing a week of the challenge, mastering a new pose, or experiencing increased comfort, acknowledge and celebrate your progress. Recognizing achievements fuels motivation and builds a positive mindset.

9. Daily Affirmations:

Start each day with a positive affirmation. Affirmations foster a positive mindset and set the tone for a day of self-care and empowerment. Consider statements that resonate with your journey, such as "I am strong," "I am resilient," or "I am deserving of well-being."

10. Supportive Resources:

Access supportive resources, including video demonstrations, written guides, and tips for adapting poses. These resources provide additional guidance and ensure you feel confident and empowered throughout the challenge.

As you embark on this 30-day Chair Yoga Challenge, remember that every breath, every movement, and every moment of mindfulness contributes to your journey of empowerment. May this structured challenge serve as a beacon of inspiration, guiding you toward a renewed sense of strength, comfort, and joy in the beautiful tapestry of your Fibromyalgia story.

Challenges of Engaging in a Chair Yoga Routine

Engaging in a chair yoga program as a Fibromyalgia patient can bring about various challenges and opportunities for positive impact on weight management, pain relief, balance, strength, flexibility, and overall well-being.

Here's an exploration of the potential challenges and benefits associated with each aspect:

1. Weight Management:

Challenge: Fibromyalgia symptoms, including fatigue and pain, may make traditional forms of exercise difficult.

Impact: Chair yoga provides a low-impact option for physical activity, supporting weight management without placing excessive strain on the joints. Consistent practice contributes to maintaining a healthy weight.

2. Pain Relief:

Challenge: Chronic pain is a central aspect of Fibromyalgia, making certain movements and exercises challenging.

Impact: Chair yoga incorporates gentle movements and modifications, offering a therapeutic approach to managing pain. Regular practice may contribute to reducing pain levels and improving overall comfort.

3. Balance:

Challenge: Fibromyalgia can affect balance and coordination, increasing the risk of falls.

Impact: Chair yoga includes poses to enhance balance, promoting stability and reducing the risk of falls. Improved balance contributes to a safer and more confident engagement in daily activities.

4. Strength:

Challenge: Muscle weakness and fatigue are common in Fibromyalgia, making strength-building exercises challenging.

Impact: Chair yoga gradually introduces strength-building poses, allowing individuals to build muscle in a controlled and accessible manner. Improved strength supports better posture and resilience against daily physical demands.

5. Flexibility:

Challenge: Stiffness and reduced range of motion are prevalent in Fibromyalgia.

Impact: Chair yoga focuses on gentle stretching and flexibility, promoting joint mobility and reducing stiffness. Increased flexibility contributes to a greater range of motion and enhanced overall comfort.

6. Overall Well-being:

Challenge: Fibromyalgia often impacts mental health, contributing to stress and fatigue.

Impact: Chair yoga incorporates mindfulness and relaxation techniques, fostering a positive impact on mental well-being. The practice encourages stress reduction, improved mood, and a sense of overall calm.

Setting Personal Goals for the Challenge

Embarking on this chair yoga challenge offers a unique opportunity to tailor the experience to your needs and aspirations. As you step into this transformative journey, I encourage you to set personal goals that resonate with your Fibromyalgia journey.

Here's a guide to help you define objectives that will empower and uplift you:

1. Reflect on Your Needs:

Begin by reflecting on your current state of well-being. Consider areas of your life affected by Fibromyalgia, whether it's pain, fatigue, stress, or specific physical limitations. Acknowledge the unique challenges you face.

2. Identify Aspects to Improve:

Pinpoint specific aspects you wish to improve or manage better during the challenge. This could include pain levels, flexibility, mood, or factors related to daily activities. Be specific in identifying areas where positive change is desired.

3. Realistic and Attainable:

Set goals that are realistic and attainable within the context of your Fibromyalgia. While challenges are meant to stretch you, they should also be within what you can reasonably achieve. This ensures a sense of accomplishment and motivation.

4. Prioritize Self-Care:

Consider how your goals align with your overall self-care. Focus on objectives contributing to your physical, mental, and emotional well-being. Prioritizing self-care reinforces a holistic approach to managing Fibromyalgia.

5. Gradual Progression:

Embrace the idea of gradual progression. Your goals can be approached incrementally, allowing for adaptation and growth throughout the challenge. Progress may be made with little, regular effort.

Examples of Personal Goals:

- **Pain Management:** "Reduce daily pain levels by incorporating chair yoga practices targeting specific pain points."
- **Flexibility:** "Improve overall flexibility and joint mobility, focusing on areas of stiffness and discomfort."
- **Stress Reduction:** "To alleviate stress and promote a feeling of calm and relaxation, consider integrating mindfulness techniques into your routine."
- **Consistent Practice:** "Establish a routine of practicing chair yoga at least three times a week to build consistency and habit."
- **Balance Enhancement:** Practice balance poses to improve stability and prevent falls during daily activities.
- **Mood Improvement:** "Use chair yoga as a tool to uplift mood and cultivate a positive mindset amidst the challenges of Fibromyalgia."

Remember:

- Your goals are personal, and they evolve as your journey progresses.
- Celebrate each milestone, recognizing your progress, no matter how small.
- Be kind to yourself. Fibromyalgia is a complex condition; your effort is a testament to your strength.

As you define your objectives for this chair yoga challenge, envision the positive impact they can have on your Fibromyalgia journey. You are setting goals and shaping a path toward greater well-being, resilience, and empowerment.

Daily Chair Yoga Routines for the Challenge

Day 1-5: Foundation and Mindful Start

Day 1:

Seated Mountain Pose (5 mins):

- Sit tall, breathe deeply, reaching arms overhead.

Neck Stretches (3 mins):

- Tilt your head gently from side to side, forward, and back.

Seated Forward Bend (5 mins):

- Hinge at hips, reach towards feet, hold.

Mindful Breathing (5 mins):

- Focus on deep, intentional breaths.

Daily Intention Setting (5 mins):

- Reflect on goals and set a positive intention.

Day 2-5:

Repeat the Day 1 routine, gradually increasing hold times.

Day 6-10: Flexibility and Gentle Stretching

Day 6:

Seated Cat-Cow Stretch (5 mins):

- Inhale (Cow), exhale (Cat), repeat.

Gentle Twist (3 mins):

- Inhale, lengthen your spine, exhale, and twist.

Seated Side Stretch (5 mins):

- Inhale, lift arms, exhale, lean to the side.

Leg Extensions (5 mins):

- Extend one leg at a time, flex, and point.

Mindful Relaxation (7 mins):

- Lie back and focus on slow breaths.

Day 7-10:

Repeat the Day 6 routine, gradually increasing hold times.

Day 11-15: Balance and Stability

Day 11:

Seated Tree Pose (5 mins):

- Lift one foot, find balance, switch.

Seated Knee Lifts (5 mins):

- Lift one knee at a time and engage the core.

Chair Squats (7 mins):

- Stand, lower into a squat, repeat.

Seated Warrior Pose (5 mins):

- Extend your leg and reach your arms overhead.

Mindful Balancing Breath (5 mins):

- Sit comfortably and focus on Breathing.

Day 12-15:

Repeat the Day 11 routine, gradually increasing hold times.

Day 16-20: Strength and Endurance Building

Day 16:

Seated Leg Lifts (7 mins):

- Lift and lower each leg, and engage the core.

Seated Arm Raises (5 mins):

- Inhale, raise arms overhead, exhale down.

Chair Plank (10 mins):

- Place hands on a chair and engage the core.

Seated Row (7 mins):

- Extend arms, pull back, squeeze shoulder blades.

Mindful Strength Meditation (5 mins):

- Visualize inner strength, meditate.

Day 17-20:

Repeat the Day 16 routine, gradually increasing reps.

Day 21-25: Pain Relief and Stress Reduction

Day 21:

Seated Child's Pose (7 mins):

- Sit back, reach your arms forward, and breathe.

Neck and Shoulder Release (5 mins):

- Roll shoulders, drop ear to shoulder.

Seated Butterfly Stretch (7 mins):

- Soles of feet together, flap knees.

Chair Pigeon Pose (5 mins):

- Cross the ankle over the knee and feel the stretch.

Guided Stress Reduction (10 mins):

- Listen to a guided meditation.

Day 22-25:

Repeat the Day 21 routine, gradually increasing hold times.

Day 26-30: Integration and Reflection

Day 26:

Complete Chair Yoga Routine (15 mins):

- Integrate poses into a whole routine.

Mindful Reflection (10 mins):

- Reflect on the 30-day journey.

Setting Future Intentions (7 mins):

- Define future well-being goals.

Day 27-30:

Repeat the Day 26 routine, emphasizing mindfulness.

Note:

- Consistency is key. Perform these routines daily or as per your comfort level.
- Adapt as needed. Listen to your body modify poses if required.
- Celebrate progress. Acknowledge achievements and milestones.
- Stay mindful. Incorporate breath awareness in each routine.

This detailed breakdown offers a structured plan for each day of the 30-Day Chair Yoga Challenge, focusing on adapting to Fibromyalgia's unique needs. Change the length and intensity based on your comfort level, advancing progressively as your body permits.

Engaging different aspects of well-being As a Fibromyaglia Patient

Understanding the diverse aspects of well-being, we embark on a journey emphasizing variety. Incorporating a diverse range of chair yoga poses and practices is not only essential for keeping the routines engaging. Still, it is also a powerful strategy for addressing various dimensions of your well-being.

Let's explore the significance of variety in chair yoga, tailored specifically for individuals managing Fibromyalgia:

1. Physical Variety:

Different Pose Categories:

- Incorporate seated, standing, and reclined poses to engage various muscle groups.
- Rotate through categories like stretches, strength-building, and balance poses.

Varied Intensity Levels:

- Alternate between gentle stretches and slightly more challenging poses.
- Gradually introduce variations to keep your body adaptable and responsive.

2. Emotional and Mental Variety:

Mindfulness Practices:

- Include mindfulness meditation and deep-breathing exercises to promote mental clarity and emotional balance.
- Experiment with guided visualizations to foster a positive mindset.

Stress Reduction Techniques:

- Integrate stress-relief practices such as progressive muscle relaxation.
- Experiment with different relaxation techniques to discover what resonates best with you.

3. Variety in Duration:

Short and Long Sessions:

- Some days, opt for more straightforward chair yoga sessions when time is limited.
- Reserve certain days for longer, more immersive practices for a comprehensive experience.

Frequent Breaks:

- Incorporate short breaks throughout the day with quick chair yoga stretches.
- This not only adds variety but also prevents monotony and stiffness.

4. Social and Community Variety:

Online Classes and Communities:

- Join online chair yoga classes to experience different teaching styles and approaches.
- Engage with online communities to share experiences and gain insights from others.

In-Person Sessions:

- Attend local chair yoga sessions, workshops, or support groups.
- The social aspect adds a dynamic element to your well-being routine.

Incorporating Tools and Props:

Chair Variations:

- Utilize different types of chairs for added variety.
- Experiment with seated poses using a stability ball or cushion.

Props for Support:

- Integrate props like bolsters, straps, or blankets for added comfort.

- Reinforcements provide variations that cater to individual needs.

5. Exploration of Breathing Techniques:

Alternate Nostril Breathing:

- Explore Nadi Shodhana (alternate nostril breathing) for a calming effect.
- Experiment with different breath ratios to find what suits your energy levels.

Breath of Fire:

- Try Kapalabhati (Breath of Fire) for an invigorating practice.
- Adjust the pace to your comfort, focusing on the cleansing nature of the breath.

Personalized Modifications:

Adapting Poses:

- Modify poses based on how you feel on any given day.

- Personalize your routine to address specific areas of concern or focus on your strengths.

Individualized Challenges:

- Set personal challenges within your practice, such as holding a pose for an extended duration.
- Adjust the challenge level based on your current abilities.

In embracing variety, acknowledge the uniqueness of your Fibromyalgia journey. This approach ensures that chair yoga becomes a dynamic and evolving part of your daily life, catering to the diverse needs of your physical, emotional, and mental well-being.

Remember, variety keeps things interesting and allows for a holistic and adaptive approach to your chair yoga practice. Embrace the diversity, and may each day bring a new facet of well-being into your journey.

Tracking progress and celebrating milestones

Embarking on the 30-Day Chair Yoga Challenge is a significant step towards holistic well-being. Tracking your progress and celebrating milestones is not just a reflection of achievements but a powerful motivator to propel you forward.

Here's a guide tailored for you, incorporating tools and methods to track your daily practice and celebrate the victories along the way:

Tracking Daily Practice:

1. Chair Yoga Journal:

Tool: Maintain a dedicated journal for your chair yoga journey.

Method: Record daily practices, noting the duration, specific poses, and any modifications.

Benefits: Provides a tangible record of your efforts and allows for self-reflection.

2. Digital Apps and Trackers:

Tool: Utilize fitness apps or habit-tracking apps.

Method: Set daily reminders and log your chair yoga sessions.

Benefits: Offers a visual representation of your consistency and progress over time.

3. Visual Calendar:

Tool: Use a large calendar or planner.

Method: Mark each day with a symbol or color to represent completed chair yoga sessions.

Benefits: Provides a quick overview of your commitment and consistency.

4. Progress Photos or Videos:

Tool: Smartphone or camera.

Method: Take photos or short videos of your practice at regular intervals.

Benefits: Visual evidence of your physical progress and improvement in poses.

5. Well-being Checklist:

Tool: Create a checklist for various aspects of well-being.

Method: Include elements like mood, energy levels, and pain perception.

Benefits: It lets you observe correlations between chair yoga and overall well-being.

Celebrating Achievements and Milestones

1. Daily Reflections:

Method: Spend a few moments each day reflecting on your practice.

Celebration: Acknowledge the effort you put in, even on challenging days.

2. Weekly Milestones:

Method: Set weekly goals and milestones.

Celebration: Treat yourself to a small reward or a moment of relaxation when achieving weekly objectives.

3. Community Sharing:

Method: Engage with online chair yoga communities.

Celebration: Share your achievements, inspire others, and receive support.

4. Reward System:

Method: Establish a reward system for achieving specific targets.

Celebration: Treat yourself to something special when reaching a predetermined milestone.

5. Personalized Incentives:

Method: Identify personal incentives that resonate with you.

Celebration: Whether it's a favorite activity, a special meal, or a moment of self-care, indulge when you hit a significant milestone.

6. Reflection Journal:

Method: Dedicate a section of your journal for reflections.

Celebration: Write down moments of triumph, gratitude, and pride in overcoming challenges.

7. Virtual or Physical Certificates:

Method: Create or find virtual or physical certificates.

Celebration: Award yourself certificates for completing specific phases or achieving set goals.

Before we call it a wrap up, meet Sarah, a resilient soul navigating the complexities of life with Fibromyalgia. Faced with daily challenges, she embarked on a 30-day chair yoga challenge to reclaim control over her well-being. Little did she know that this decision would lead to a transformative experience.

In the initial days, Sarah focused on foundational poses, adapting them to her unique needs. She found solace in the Seated Mountain Pose and gentle stretches, gradually building her practice. Despite initial doubts, Sarah noticed a subtle shift in her energy levels and a newfound sense of calm.

As Sarah delved deeper into the challenge, she began exploring more diverse poses. The combination of flexibility, balance, and strength-building exercises brought a breakthrough. Sarah's pain levels diminished, and she experienced enhanced flexibility, a testament to the adaptability of chair yoga.

By the final week, Sarah had become a chair yoga enthusiast. She seamlessly flowed through a complete routine, effortlessly transitioning between poses. Sarah's sleep improved, and she woke up with a vitality that had long eluded her. Her journey became an inspiring testament to the power of consistency and self-care.

As we conclude this chapter, let Sarah's journey serve as a beacon of hope and encouragement. In just 30 days, she witnessed transformative results, breaking free from the limitations imposed by Fibromyalgia.

Sarah's story is not a mere anecdote; it's a testament to the potential for positive change within reach. The 30-day chair yoga challenge is not just a routine; it's a catalyst for transformation. In embracing this challenge, you are not merely committing to physical movements but opening the door to a journey that can profoundly impact your well-being.

In just 30 days, you can experience increased flexibility, reduced pain, and a newfound sense of balance. Daily commitment can bring clarity to your mind, alleviate stress, and foster a positive mindset. As Sarah discovered, the journey is not solely about physical poses; it's about reclaiming control over your narrative and fostering resilience.

Acknowledge the effort you put into each practice, regardless of the scale. Celebrate the small triumphs – the ease of a stretch, the peacefulness of a breath, and the resilience to show up daily.

Your journey is uniquely yours. What works for you may differ from others, and that's perfectly okay. Be patient and compassionate with yourself, understanding that positive change unfolds at its own pace.

As you embrace this challenge, visualize the potential for positive change in 30 days. Your commitment to yourself is a profound act of self-love and resilience. You're not just practicing chair yoga but investing in your well-being, one day at a time.

Conclusion

As we conclude this 30-day chair yoga challenge, it's a moment to pause, reflect, and celebrate your remarkable journey. This venture into mindful movement has been more than just a series of poses; it's been a profound exploration of self-care and well-being.

In 30 days, you've engaged in physical movements and embarked on a journey of self-discovery. You've cultivated a deeper connection between your mind and body through chair yoga. The awareness of breath, the gentle stretches, and the intentional movements have harmonized to create a sense of unity.

You've witnessed the remarkable adaptability of chair yoga, tailor-made for your unique needs. Your resilience in overcoming daily challenges, whether physical or mental, reflects the strength within you. Incorporating mindfulness practices has been a beacon of calm amid life's storms.

By practicing chair yoga, you've woven moments of serenity into your daily routine, reducing stress and fostering a tranquil mindset.

Notice the improvements in your physical well-being – increased flexibility, reduced pain, and a general sense of vitality. Acknowledge the emotional benefits, from enhanced mood to a more positive outlook.

Your commitment to this challenge has demonstrated the power of character. By showing up daily, you've formed a habit and laid the foundation for lasting positive change. As we bid farewell to the formal structure of this challenge, let this not be an end but a transition. Chair yoga need not be confined to a set timeframe; it can become a constant companion in your journey toward well-being.

Let chair yoga seamlessly integrate into your daily routine, becoming a self-care ritual. Whether it's a five-minute stretch in the morning or an evening wind-down, let it be a consistent part of your life. Feel empowered to personalize your chair yoga practice based on your needs and preferences.

Experiment with poses, durations, and mindfulness techniques to create an approach that resonates with you. Take the principles of mindful movement beyond the chair into your everyday life.

Cultivate awareness in daily activities, bringing the spirit of mindfulness into each moment.

I extend heartfelt gratitude to you for your dedication and commitment throughout this 30-day mindful movement journey. Your commitment to daily practice is a testament to your resilience and self-care.

Reflect on your physical and mental progress, whether it's improved flexibility, reduced pain, or a heightened sense of well-being. Express gratitude to yourself for prioritizing your well-being and embarking on this transformative journey.

Let's carry forward the positive energy cultivated during this challenge in the spirit of celebration. Your mindful movement journey is an ongoing story, and each day is a new opportunity for growth, self-discovery, and well-being.

BONUS CHAPTER:

Mindful Living Beyond the Mat

Have you ever thought about the impact chair yoga could have on your day-to-day routines? It's more than just a form of exercise; it's a philosophy that extends beyond the physical aspects of the practice. The chair becomes a tool for bringing mindfulness into different parts of your life.

Chair yoga goes beyond being a set of postures; it embodies more profound principles that extend beyond the mat. We aim to understand these principles and see how they can naturally integrate into your daily life.

As we move forward, we'll touch on concepts like mindfulness, balance, and tranquility embedded in chair yoga. These principles can contribute to your physical well-being and shape how you interact with the world. It's a journey that goes beyond the routine, prompting you to embrace mindful living in every breath and every moment.

In our upcoming discussion, we'll explore self-awareness and how chair yoga can transform your daily rituals. The chair, often considered a simple object, becomes a catalyst for introspection, providing a space where the synergy of your body and mind unfolds.

Think about the saying, "Mindful Living Beyond the Mat." It makes us wonder: Can the calm feeling on a yoga mat go beyond that space and be part of our daily life? This question is about thinking and doing practical things. It's like asking if we can take the good feelings from yoga and use them in everyday life.

Chair yoga means doing it while sitting on a chair, not just on a mat. This kind of yoga goes beyond what we usually think of—bending and breathing. It's about being aware and calm in everyday activities, like sitting in a chair. The chair we often use becomes a way to bring yoga ideas into our daily lives.

The point is not just to keep yoga on the mat but to use its intelligent ideas in all parts of our lives. Exploring chair yoga means going on a journey where awareness is essential, not just when doing yoga poses but also in how we think and feel daily.

Imagine a regular day—going to work, doing your job, or just taking a break by sitting. Chair yoga suggests we should pay attention in these normal times. We should be mindful—meaning we deliberately think about our mind, body, and breathing. The smooth movements in yoga poses can be similar to how we gracefully do our daily tasks, making everyday things more meaningful.

Also, thinking about "Mindful Living Beyond the Mat" means considering how chair yoga affects our well-being in general. It asks us to see how yoga ideas like balance, focus, and calmness can improve our relationships, clear our thoughts, and make us feel healthy in all parts of our lives.

Ultimately, "Mindful Living Beyond the Mat" is like an invitation to go beyond just doing yoga on a mat. It suggests bringing the good parts of yoga into all aspects of our daily lives, especially when we're just sitting in a chair. It's like discovering the great possibilities inside us and making a harmonious balance of our mind, body, and feelings in everything we do.

Incorporating Mindfulness into Daily Activities

First off, imagine making your everyday activities more than just routines. You know, like turning the mundane stuff into moments of mindfulness. It's easier than it sounds. You can try little techniques to sprinkle mindfulness into your day—whether sipping your morning coffee, walking, or doing chores.

These techniques aren't about adding more stress to your day. Instead, they're like minor tweaks that make your routine moments more memorable. For example, feel the warmth in your hands when sipping that coffee, savor the taste, and be there in the moment. It's like turning an ordinary coffee break into a mini vacation for your mind.

Now, let's talk about the transformative power of being aware. It's like giving yourself a superpower for feeling good. Cultivating awareness is about paying attention to what's happening around and inside you. When you're aware, it's like turning on a light in a dark room—you see things more clearly.

This awareness isn't just about the big stuff; it's in the little details, too. Like feeling the ground beneath your feet as you walk or tasting the flavors in your food. It's about being present in the now and soaking up the goodness of each moment.

So, when we talk about the holistic application of mindfulness and movement, it's saying, "Hey, let's make feeling good a whole-life thing." It's not just about a few minutes of meditation; it's about weaving mindfulness into everything you do, big or small.

Think of it as a recipe for sustained well-being—making your daily grind a bit more mindful, aware, and awesome. Give it a shot, and let me know how it feels!

Techniques for bringing mindfulness to everyday tasks.

Let's explore some cool ways to bring mindfulness into everyday tasks—making the ordinary feel extraordinary.

- **Slow It Down:**

Try slowing down your pace when you're doing something routine, like washing dishes or walking to work. Feel the water on your hands or notice your feet hitting the ground. Slowing down lets you savor the moment.

- **Use Your Senses:**

Pay attention to your senses during daily tasks. If you're eating, really taste the food. Feel the texture, smell the aroma. Engaging your senses brings you into the present and makes the experience richer.

- **One Thing at a Time:**

Multitasking might seem efficient, but it's different from the mindfulness MVP. Instead, focus on one task at a time. Whether it's replying to emails or folding laundry, give your full attention to each thing you do.

- **Breathe and Center:**

Take a moment to breathe. It doesn't have to be a big production—just a few deep breaths. This simple act can ground you and bring a sense of calm, even during a hectic day.

- **Mindful Listening:**

When in conversation, practice mindful listening. Put away distractions, look the person in the eyes, and absorb what they're saying. It builds connections and makes the interaction more meaningful.

- **Turn Chores into Mindful Moments:**

Chores often get a bad rap, but they can be moments of mindfulness. Whether you're folding clothes or vacuuming, focus on the task at hand. Notice the textures, colors, and movements involved.

- **Mindful Commuting:**

If you commute, turn it into a mindfulness exercise. Instead of stressing about traffic, use the time to notice your surroundings. Feel the steering wheel, listen to the sounds, and be present in the journey.

Remember, these are just ideas—feel free to get creative and find what works best for you. Bringing mindfulness into everyday tasks is like turning the ordinary into the extraordinary, one moment at a time. Give it a shot, and see how it adds sparkle to your day!

The transformative power of cultivating awareness.

Picture this: You're doing your thing, but instead of just going through the motions, awareness kicks in. It's like suddenly having a super-sharp focus on whatever you're doing—work, chatting with friends, or even just taking a stroll. It's about making everything more transparent and more vibrant.

Being aware is like turning up the quality of your interactions. It's about genuinely listening when someone's talking, understanding your thoughts and feelings, and being present in your relationships. It's the difference between just being there and connecting.

Life throws curveballs, right? But having awareness on your side is like having a stress-beating buddy. It's not about avoiding challenges; it's about facing them with a clear head and a calm attitude. It's your secret weapon against stress.

Cultivating awareness is like the magic ingredient in mindfulness.

It's about paying attention to each moment, whether it's something big or just a regular, everyday thing. It turns the mundane into something special. Awareness isn't just about the outside stuff; it's also about understanding what's happening inside you. It's like giving your emotional intelligence a significant upgrade. You become more in sync with your feelings, making navigating life's ups and downs easier.

In simple terms, cultivating awareness is like turning on the lights in a dark room. Suddenly, you see things more clearly, experience life more deeply, and handle challenges with a newfound clarity.

So, how about giving it a shot? Start by taking a moment to breathe and notice what's happening around you. It's a small step with big rewards.

Integrating chair yoga principles into dietary choices and sleep habits.

You know that chair you use daily, whether at your desk, the kitchen table, or just a comfy spot? Well, that chair can be more than just a place to sit. It can be like your own health companion.

Imagine taking a break from your usual routine and trying some easy chair yoga moves. You don't need to be a yoga expert; it's about moving a bit while sitting. You could stretch your arms, twist your torso, or take a few slow breaths. It's like giving your body a little treat in your chair. These simple moves can help ease tension, make you feel more flexible, and give you a moment to relax without leaving your seat.

So, next time you're in your chair, think of it as your health buddy, and give those chair yoga moves a shot. Your body might thank you with some good vibes Eating healthy also doesn't need to be tricky. Keep it simple—add some veggies to your meals, drink water, and enjoy your food. It's like giving your body what it needs without making it a giant puzzle.

Sleep is like a superhero for feeling good. There is no need for fancy tricks—aim for a regular sleep routine. Turn off screens before bedtime, get cozy, and let your body do its thing. It's like giving yourself a nightly recharge.

Exercise doesn't have to be a big deal. Just move a bit each day. Take a short walk, dance around a bit, or stretch. It's like telling your body, "Hey, we're active, but we're keeping it chill," it keeps everything running smoothly.

Screens are everywhere. But too much can be a bit much. Take breaks, look away, and give your eyes and brain a break. It's like finding the balance between being connected and giving yourself screen-free moments.

Water is like a magic potion for your body. Keep it accessible—sip water throughout the day. It's like a little splash of goodness that helps everything work smoothly.

Life can get busy. Take a minute to breathe. It's not complicated—just a few deep breaths. It's like hitting pause, calming your mind, and then getting back to what you're doing with a clear head.

So, these healthy ideas are all about keeping it simple. No fancy stuff—just little changes you can slide into your day. It's like building a stash of easy, feel-good tricks.

Creating a balanced and sustainable lifestyle.

Building a balanced and sustainable lifestyle is like creating harmony between different aspects of your life to keep it going in the long run. It's about finding a sweet spot that works for you physically, mentally, and emotionally.

1. Balanced Diet:

Eating a mix of different foods is the key. Include fruits, veggies, whole grains, and proteins. There is no need for extreme diets—aim for a variety that satisfies your taste buds and gives your body what it needs.

2. Regular Exercise:

You don't need to run a marathon, but you must move your body regularly. It could be a daily walk, home workouts, or activities you enjoy. The idea is to keep things active without overwhelming yourself.

3. Quality Sleep:

Your body needs good sleep to recharge. Set a consistent sleep schedule, create a comfy sleep environment, and wind down before bedtime. It's like giving your body a chance to refresh and prepare for a new day.

4. Stress Management:

Life can get hectic, so find what helps you chill out. It might be deep breaths, a hobby you enjoy, or spending time with loved ones. Managing stress is like maintaining a calm sea amid life's storms.

5. Time for Yourself:

Amidst all the hustle, carve out some "me time." It could be reading, listening to music, or just sitting quietly. It's like recharging your batteries and balancing between doing things for yourself and others.

6. Stay Hydrated:

Water is your best friend. Keep it simple—sip water throughout the day. It helps with digestion, energy levels, and overall well-being. It's like giving your body a daily dose of freshness.

7. Set Realistic Goals:

Aim for achievable goals that align with your values. Whether it's work, personal growth, or relationships, set realistic expectations. It's like building a bridge to success step by step.

8. Connect with Others:

Relationships matter. Spend time with friends and family. It's like nurturing the roots that keep you grounded and supported.

Remember, it's not about perfection but finding what works for you and making small, sustainable changes. Building a balanced lifestyle is a journey, not a destination. Enjoy the process and create a life that's not just lived but truly enjoyed!

Mindful Stress Management

Imagine this: You're facing a challenging moment and have a chair nearby. Well, that chair can be your ally in stress relief. Try some easy chair yoga moves—simple stretches, a gentle twist, or just taking a moment to breathe. It's like giving your body and mind a timeout in your chair. These quick exercises can help ease tension and bring a sense of calm when you need it most.

Now, let's connect the dots between mindfulness and mental resilience. Mindfulness is about being present in the moment, even in the face of stress. Practicing mindfulness is like having a mental shield that helps you stay strong when things get tough. It's not about avoiding stress but facing it with a clear mind and a steady spirit. By being aware of your thoughts and feelings without getting overwhelmed, you build mental resilience—it's like having a solid foundation to weather life's ups and downs.

So, next time stress knocks on your door, consider turning to your chair yoga moves and embracing mindfulness. It's a simple yet powerful combo that helps you navigate challenging moments more easily.

Chair yoga techniques for stress relief during challenging moments.

1: Seated Forward Bend

- Sit comfortably on your chair with your feet flat on the floor.
- Take a deep breath and lengthen your spine.
- Hinge at your hips, leaning forward.
- Allow your arms to hang down or reach toward the floor.
- Hold for a few breaths to release tension in your back and shoulders.

2: Neck and Shoulder Release

- While sitting, drop your right ear towards your right shoulder.
- Hold for a few breaths, feeling a stretch on the left side of your neck.
- Switch to the other side.
- Add a gentle neck roll, moving your head in a circular motion to release tension.

3: Seated Cat-Cow Stretch

- Sit at the edge of your chair with your hands on your knees.
- Inhale as you arch your back, lifting your chest and looking up (Cow Pose).
- Exhale as you round your back, tucking your chin to your chest (Cat Pose).
- Repeat these movements, syncing them with your breath.

4: Deep Breathing

- Sit comfortably, close your eyes, and focus on your breath.
- Inhale deeply through your nose, allowing your belly to expand.
- Exhale slowly through your mouth.
- Repeat several times to calm the nervous system and induce relaxation.

5: Seated Twist

- While sitting, turn your upper body to the right.

- Hold onto the back of your chair for support.
- Hold for a few breaths, feeling the stretch along your spine.
- Repeat on the other side to release tension and promote renewal.

6: Mindful Meditation

- Sit comfortably, close your eyes, and pay attention to your breathing.
- Inhale deeply, exhale slowly.
- Acknowledge thoughts without judgment, bringing focus back to your breath.
- Practice this mindfulness meditation for clarity and calmness.

Feel free to customize the order or repeat any step as needed. These chair yoga techniques can be your go-to stress relief routine when facing challenging moments.

The connection between mindfulness and mental resilience.

Understanding the connection between mindfulness and mental resilience is like uncovering a powerful partnership that helps us navigate life's challenges with strength and clarity.

1. Awareness in the Present Moment:

Mindfulness is all about being present in the here and now. It's like shining a light on the current moment without being overly consumed by the past or anxious about the future. This awareness provides a stable foundation, allowing us to face challenges one moment at a time.

2. Acknowledging and Accepting Thoughts and Emotions:

Instead of pushing away or getting overwhelmed by complex thoughts and emotions, mindfulness encourages acknowledgment and acceptance. It's like saying, "Okay, I feel this way, and that's alright." This non-judgmental attitude fosters a sense of resilience by allowing us to respond to challenges with a clear mind.

3. Building Emotional Regulation:

Mindfulness helps us regulate our emotions by giving us the space to observe and understand them. It's like having a pause button—allowing us to respond thoughtfully rather than impulsively. This emotional regulation is crucial to mental resilience, helping us bounce back from setbacks.

4. Stress Reduction and Cortisol Regulation:

Regular mindfulness practices have been linked to reduced stress levels and better regulation of cortisol, the stress hormone. It's like having a built-in stress management system. By keeping stress in check, mindfulness contributes to our mental resilience, helping us stay composed in the face of adversity.

5. Enhancing Cognitive Flexibility:

Mindfulness encourages an open and flexible mindset. It's like widening the lens through which we view challenges. This cognitive flexibility allows us to adapt to changing situations, find alternative solutions, and see possibilities even under challenging circumstances—hallmarks of mental resilience.

6. Improved Focus and Concentration:

Practicing mindfulness sharpens our focus and concentration. It's like training the mind to stay on task amidst distractions. This enhanced focus enables us to tackle challenges with a clearer mind, contributing to our ability to endure and overcome difficulties.

7. Cultivating a Non-Attached Perspective:

Mindfulness teaches us to observe our thoughts and emotions without becoming overly attached. It's like watching clouds pass by without being swept away. This non-attached perspective fosters resilience by preventing us from being overwhelmed or defined by challenging experiences.

8. Strengthening Mind-Body Connection:

The mind and body are closely connected. Mindfulness practices, such as mindful breathing, promote this connection. It's like syncing the mind and body in a harmonious dance. This connection contributes to overall well-being and resilience by ensuring that both aspects of our being work together efficiently.

In essence, mindfulness and mental resilience go hand in hand. Mindfulness provides the tools and mindset to face challenges with composure, adaptability, and a clear sense of self. It's not about avoiding difficulties but facing them with a resilient spirit and a grounded mind.
Chair yoga transcends physical postures, offering a versatile tool for a mindful lifestyle. Accessible anywhere with a chair, it requires no fancy equipment. Its emphasis on intentional breathing becomes a powerful stress antidote, fostering calm amid daily chaos. Chair yoga harmonizes body and mind, cultivating balance in both.

The resilience built extends beyond sessions, aiding composure in life's challenges. Integrating it into daily rituals seamlessly weaves mindfulness into your lifestyle. Are you ready for this transformative journey?

Made in the USA
Columbia, SC
09 July 2025

60555677R00157